CKD STAGE 4 COOKBOOK FOR SENIORS

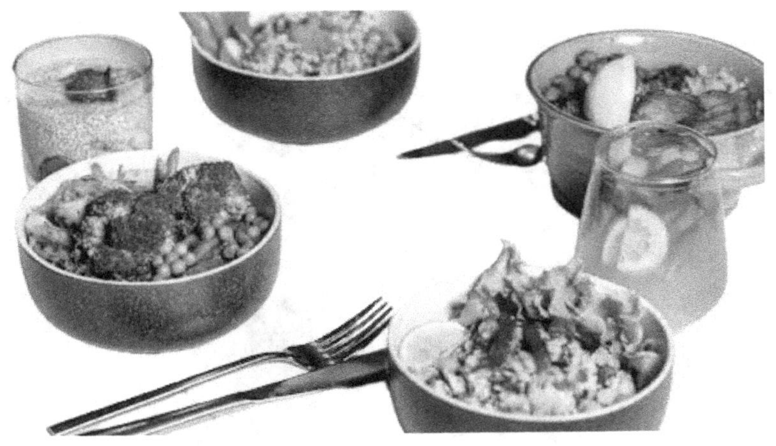

DR. VICKIE STOCK

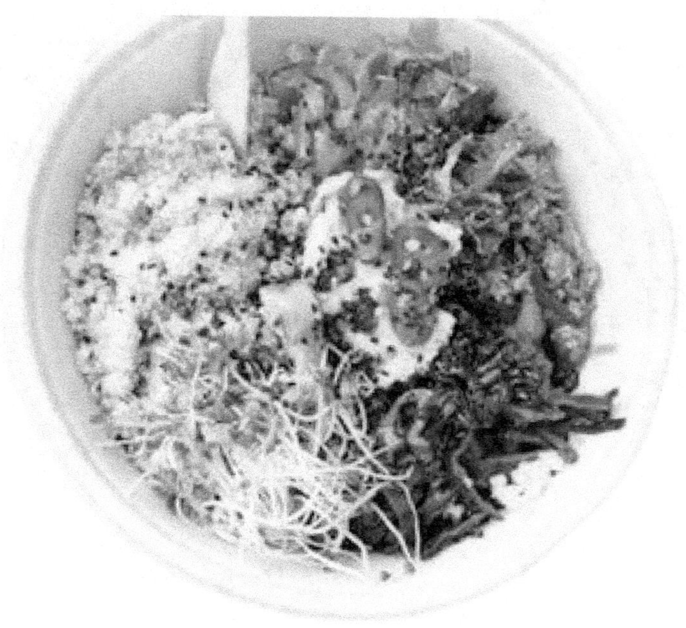

TABLE OF CONTENT

CHAPTER ONE: Understanding CKD Stage 4

Chronic Kidney Disease (CKD) is a progressive condition characterized by the gradual loss of kidney function over time. In stage 4 of CKD, kidney function is significantly impaired, with the glomerular filtration rate (GFR) ranging from 15 to 29 milliliters per minute per 1.73 square meters.

This stage is often referred to as advanced kidney disease or severe reduction in kidney function. Understanding the overview of CKD stage 4 is crucial for individuals affected by this condition, as well as their caregivers and healthcare providers.

In CKD stage 4, the kidneys are unable to effectively filter waste products and excess fluids from the blood, leading to a buildup of toxins and fluid retention in the body.

As kidney function declines, individuals may experience symptoms such as fatigue, weakness, swelling in the legs and ankles, shortness of breath, and difficulty concentrating.

Complications of CKD stage 4 can include high blood pressure, anemia, bone disease, electrolyte imbalances, and cardiovascular disease. Management of CKD stage 4 focuses on slowing the progression of kidney damage, managing symptoms, and preventing complications. This often involves a combination of lifestyle modifications, medication therapy, and close monitoring by healthcare professionals. Dietary changes, such as limiting sodium, phosphorus, and potassium intake, may be necessary to reduce strain on the kidneys and maintain overall health.

Regular monitoring of kidney function through blood tests, urine tests, and imaging studies is essential for managing CKD stage 4 and adjusting treatment as needed. In some cases, individuals with advanced kidney disease may require dialysis or kidney transplantation to sustain life.

Overall, CKD stage 4 is a serious and potentially life-threatening condition that requires ongoing management and support. By understanding the overview of CKD stage 4 and working closely with healthcare providers, individuals can take proactive steps to optimize their health and quality of life despite the challenges posed by advanced kidney disease.

Symptoms and Complications

Symptoms and complications of Chronic Kidney Disease (CKD) stage 4 can significantly impact an individual's quality of life and overall health. As kidney function declines, various physiological processes in the body are disrupted, leading to a range of symptoms and potential complications.

Symptoms of CKD stage 4 often become more pronounced as kidney function decreases. Common symptoms include fatigue, weakness, and a general feeling of malaise. Individuals may also experience swelling in the legs and ankles, known as edema, due to fluid retention caused by impaired kidney function.

Other symptoms can include shortness of breath, difficulty concentrating, decreased appetite, and changes in urinary habits, such as increased frequency or decreased urine output.

Complications of CKD stage 4 can affect multiple organ systems and have serious consequences for overall health. One common complication is high blood pressure (hypertension), which can further damage the kidneys and increase the risk of cardiovascular events such as heart attack and stroke.

Anemia is another common complication of CKD, resulting from decreased production of red blood cells by the kidneys. Anemia can cause fatigue, weakness, and shortness of breath, further impacting quality of life.

Bone disease, characterized by weakened bones and an increased risk of fractures, is also a complication of CKD stage 4. This occurs due to abnormalities in mineral metabolism and impaired production of vitamin D by the kidneys. Additionally, electrolyte imbalances, such as hyperkalemia (elevated potassium levels) and metabolic acidosis (excess acid in the blood), can lead to muscle weakness, cardiac arrhythmias, and other complications.

Other potential complications of CKD stage 4 include fluid overload, which can result in congestive heart failure and pulmonary edema, as well as impaired immune function, increasing susceptibility to infections. Neurological complications, such as peripheral neuropathy and cognitive impairment, may also occur as a result of CKD-related changes in nerve function.

Overall, recognizing and managing symptoms and complications of CKD stage 4 are essential for preserving kidney function, reducing the risk of complications, and improving quality of life for affected individuals. Close monitoring by healthcare providers and adherence to treatment recommendations are crucial for optimizing outcomes in individuals with advanced kidney disease.

Importance of Nutrition in CKD Management

The importance of nutrition in the management of Chronic Kidney Disease (CKD) cannot be overstated, particularly in stage 4 where kidney function is significantly impaired.

A well-planned diet plays a vital role in slowing the progression of kidney damage, managing symptoms, and preventing complications associated with CKD.

One of the primary goals of nutrition therapy in CKD stage 4 is to reduce the workload on the kidneys by limiting the intake of certain nutrients, such as sodium, phosphorus, and potassium.

Excess sodium can lead to fluid retention and high blood pressure, both of which can exacerbate kidney damage and increase the risk of cardiovascular events.

Phosphorus and potassium are electrolytes that can accumulate in the blood when kidney function is impaired, leading to imbalances that can affect bone health, muscle function, and heart rhythm.

Another key aspect of nutrition therapy in CKD stage 4 is ensuring an adequate intake of high-quality protein while limiting proteinuria (protein in the urine).

Protein is essential for maintaining muscle mass and supporting overall health, but excessive protein intake can increase the burden on the kidneys. Therefore, individuals with CKD are often advised to follow a moderate protein diet, focusing on lean sources of protein such as poultry, fish, eggs, and plant-based sources like beans and tofu.

In addition to controlling nutrient intake, nutrition therapy in CKD stage 4 aims to optimize overall dietary patterns to promote health and well-being. This may involve increasing consumption of fruits, vegetables, whole grains, and healthy fats while limiting processed foods, sugary beverages, and saturated fats. Adequate hydration is also crucial for individuals with CKD to help maintain fluid balance and support kidney function.

Individualized nutrition counseling by a registered dietitian is essential for developing a tailored dietary plan that meets the specific needs and preferences of each individual with CKD stage 4. Regular monitoring of nutritional status, blood chemistry, and kidney function is necessary to assess the effectiveness of nutrition therapy and make adjustments as needed.

Overall, adopting a kidney-friendly diet and making healthy food choices can significantly improve outcomes and quality of life for individuals with CKD stage 4. By working closely with healthcare providers and adhering to dietary recommendations, individuals can take proactive steps to support kidney health and overall well-being.

CHAPTER TWO: Tip for Managing CKD Stage 4

Lifestyle Modifications

Lifestyle modifications are a critical component of managing Chronic Kidney Disease (CKD) stage 4, as they can help slow the progression of kidney damage, alleviate symptoms, and reduce the risk of complications. Several key lifestyle changes can positively impact kidney health and overall well-being in individuals with CKD.

Healthy Diet: Adopting a kidney-friendly diet is essential for individuals with CKD stage 4. This typically involves reducing sodium, phosphorus, and potassium intake while ensuring an adequate intake of high-quality protein and nutrient-rich foods.

Following a balanced diet that includes plenty of fruits, vegetables, whole grains, and lean proteins can help support kidney function and promote overall health.

Regular Exercise: Engaging in regular physical activity can have numerous benefits for individuals with CKD stage 4, including improved cardiovascular health, weight management, and increased energy levels. Exercise can also help lower blood pressure, reduce inflammation, and improve insulin sensitivity, all of which are important for managing CKD and reducing the risk of complications.

Smoking Cessation: Smoking is a major risk factor for kidney disease progression and cardiovascular complications in individuals with CKD. Quitting smoking can significantly improve kidney health and overall health outcomes.

Healthcare providers can provide support and resources to help individuals quit smoking, such as counseling, nicotine replacement therapy, and prescription medications.

Stress Management: Chronic stress can exacerbate symptoms and complications of CKD, such as high blood pressure and inflammation. Practicing stress-reducing techniques such as mindfulness meditation, deep breathing exercises, and yoga can help individuals manage stress and improve overall well-being.

Maintaining a Healthy Weight: Achieving and maintaining a healthy weight is important for individuals with CKD stage 4, as obesity can contribute to hypertension, diabetes, and cardiovascular disease, all of which can worsen kidney function. Adopting a healthy diet and engaging in regular physical activity can help individuals achieve and maintain a healthy weight.

Medication Adherence: Following prescribed medication regimens is crucial for managing CKD stage 4 and preventing complications. Individuals should take medications as directed by their healthcare providers and communicate any concerns or side effects promptly.

Overall, lifestyle modifications such as adopting a healthy diet, engaging in regular exercise, quitting smoking, managing stress, maintaining a healthy weight, and adhering to medication regimens are essential for managing CKD stage 4 and optimizing kidney health and overall well-being. By making positive lifestyle changes, individuals can improve their quality of life and reduce the risk of complications associated with CKD.

Medication Management

Medication management is a crucial aspect of managing chronic kidney disease (CKD) stage 4, as it helps alleviate symptoms, slow disease progression, and reduce the risk of complications. Individuals with CKD stage 4 often require multiple medications to address various health concerns and optimize kidney function.

One of the primary goals of medication management in CKD stage 4 is to control blood pressure. Hypertension is a common complication of CKD and can accelerate kidney damage if left uncontrolled. Medications such as angiotensin-converting enzyme (ACE) inhibitors and angiotensin II receptor blockers (ARBs) are often prescribed to lower blood pressure and protect the kidneys from further damage.

Another important aspect of medication management in CKD stage 4 is managing electrolyte imbalances. Impaired kidney function can lead to abnormalities in potassium, phosphorus, and calcium levels, which can have serious consequences for overall health. Medications such as phosphate binders and vitamin D analogs may be prescribed to help regulate electrolyte levels and maintain bone health.

Anemia is a common complication of CKD stage 4, resulting from decreased production of red blood cells by the kidneys. Medications such as erythropoiesis-stimulating agents (ESAs) and iron supplements may be prescribed to stimulate red blood cell production and alleviate symptoms of anemia, such as fatigue and weakness.

Individuals with CKD stage 4 are also at increased risk of developing cardiovascular disease. Medications such as statins, antiplatelet agents, and anticoagulants may be prescribed to reduce the risk of heart attack, stroke, and other cardiovascular events.

In addition to managing specific complications of CKD stage 4, medication management also involves addressing comorbid conditions such as diabetes, hyperlipidemia, and acidosis.

Healthcare providers work closely with individuals with CKD stage 4 to develop individualized medication regimens that address their specific health needs while minimizing side effects and drug interactions.

Regular monitoring of kidney function, blood pressure, electrolyte levels, and medication effectiveness is essential for ensuring optimal medication management in CKD stage 4.

Individuals should communicate any concerns or changes in symptoms to their healthcare providers promptly to adjust medication regimens as needed. By effectively managing medications, individuals with CKD stage 4 can improve their quality of life and reduce the risk of complications associated with advanced kidney disease.

Monitoring Kidney Function

Monitoring kidney function is essential for individuals with Chronic Kidney Disease (CKD) stage 4 to assess disease progression, guide treatment decisions, and prevent complications.

Regular monitoring allows healthcare providers to evaluate kidney function, identify changes in kidney health, and intervene promptly to optimize outcomes. One of the primary methods used to monitor kidney function is measuring glomerular filtration rate (GFR). GFR is a measure of how well the kidneys are filtering waste products from the blood. In CKD stage 4, GFR is significantly reduced, indicating advanced kidney damage. Healthcare providers use blood tests to estimate GFR, such as serum creatinine levels, and may also use imaging tests such as ultrasound or CT scans to assess kidney structure and function.

Another important parameter monitored in CKD stage 4 is proteinuria, or the presence of protein in the urine. Proteinuria is a sign of kidney damage and can indicate progressive kidney disease. Healthcare providers may perform urine tests, such as urine dipstick or urine albumin-to-creatinine ratio (ACR), to assess proteinuria and monitor changes over time.

In addition to GFR and proteinuria, healthcare providers may monitor electrolyte levels, such as potassium, phosphorus, and calcium, to assess kidney function and guide treatment decisions. Electrolyte imbalances are common in CKD stage 4 and can have serious consequences for overall health if left uncontrolled.

Blood pressure monitoring is also essential for individuals with CKD stage 4, as hypertension is a common complication of kidney disease. Elevated blood pressure can accelerate kidney damage and increase the risk of cardiovascular events. Healthcare providers may recommend home blood pressure monitoring or ambulatory blood pressure monitoring to assess blood pressure control and adjust medications as needed.

CHAPTER THREE: Stage 4 CKD Recipes for Seniors

BREAKFAST CKD STAGE 4 RECIPES FOR SENIORS

1: Creamy Banana Oatmeal

- Ingredients:
- 1/2 cup rolled oats
- 1 ripe banana, mashed
- 1 cup unsweetened almond milk
- 1/2 teaspoon cinnamon
- 1 tablespoon chopped walnuts (optional)

Instructions:

- In a saucepan, combine the rolled oats and almond milk. Bring to a gentle boil over medium heat.
- Reduce the heat to low and simmer, stirring occasionally, for 5-7 minutes or until the oats are cooked and the mixture thickens.
- Stir in the mashed banana and cinnamon until well combined.
- Remove from heat and let it sit for a minute to thicken.
- Serve the oatmeal in bowls, garnished with chopped walnuts if desired.

- Enjoy this creamy and nutritious breakfast!

Health Benefits:

- Oats are a good source of fiber, which helps regulate blood sugar levels and promote digestive health.
- Bananas are rich in potassium and vitamin C, supporting heart health and immune function.
- Almond milk adds creaminess without adding excess phosphorus or potassium, making it suitable for individuals with CKD Stage 4.
- Cinnamon may help improve insulin sensitivity and lower blood sugar levels.

Nutritional Value (per serving):

- Calories: 250
- Protein: 6g
- Carbohydrates: 44g
- Fat: 6g
- Fiber: 7g
- Potassium: 335mg

Preparation Time: 10 minutes

2: Veggie Egg Scramble

Ingredients:

- 2 large eggs
- 1/4 cup chopped bell peppers
- 1/4 cup chopped spinach
- 1 tablespoon diced onions
- 1 teaspoon olive oil
- Salt and pepper to taste

Instructions:

- Heat olive oil in a non-stick skillet over medium heat.
- Add diced onions and sauté until translucent.
- Add chopped bell peppers and spinach to the skillet and cook until vegetables are tender.
- In a bowl, whisk the eggs with salt and pepper.
- Pour the whisked eggs into the skillet with the cooked vegetables.
- Cook, stirring gently, until the eggs are set and scrambled.
- Transfer the scrambled eggs to a plate and serve hot.
- Enjoy this protein-packed breakfast with a side of whole grain toast or fresh fruit.

Health Benefits:

- Eggs are a complete protein source, providing essential amino acids for muscle health and repair.
- Bell peppers and spinach are rich in antioxidants, vitamins, and minerals, supporting immune function and overall health.
- Olive oil adds heart-healthy fats and enhances flavor without adding excess sodium.

Nutritional Value (per serving):

- Calories: 200
- Protein: 13g
- Carbohydrates: 5g
- Fat: 15g
- Fiber: 2g
- Potassium: 200mg

Preparation Time: 15 minutes

3: Greek Yogurt Parfait

Ingredients:

- 1/2 cup low-fat Greek yogurt
- 1/4 cup sliced strawberries
- 1 tablespoon chopped almonds

- 1 tablespoon ground flaxseeds
- 1 teaspoon honey (optional)

Instructions:

- In a serving glass or bowl, layer half of the Greek yogurt.
- Top the yogurt with half of the sliced strawberries.
- Sprinkle half of the chopped almonds and ground flaxseeds over the strawberries.
- Repeat the layers with the remaining yogurt, strawberries, almonds, and flaxseeds.
- Drizzle honey on top if desired for added sweetness.
- Serve immediately and enjoy this protein-rich and fiber-filled breakfast parfait!

Health Benefits:

- Greek yogurt is a good source of protein and calcium, supporting muscle and bone health.
- Strawberries are low in potassium and high in antioxidants, vitamins, and fiber, promoting heart health and digestion.
- Almonds and flaxseeds add healthy fats and omega-3 fatty acids, which may help reduce inflammation and improve cholesterol levels.
- Honey adds natural sweetness without raising blood sugar levels significantly.

Nutritional Value (per serving):

- Calories: 200
- Protein: 15g
- Carbohydrates: 15g
- Fat: 8g
- Fiber: 5g
- Potassium: 250mg

Preparation Time: 5 minutes

4: Avocado Toast with Poached Egg

Ingredients:

- 1 slice whole grain bread
- 1/4 ripe avocado, mashed
- 1 large egg
- Salt and pepper to taste
- Fresh herbs (such as parsley or chives) for garnish (optional)

Instructions:

- Toast the whole grain bread until golden brown.
- Spread the mashed avocado evenly on top of the toast.
- In a small saucepan, bring water to a simmer.
- Crack the egg into a small bowl and carefully slide it into the simmering water.

- Poach the egg for 3-4 minutes or until the whites are set but the yolk is still runny.
- Using a slotted spoon, carefully remove the poached egg from the water and place it on top of the avocado toast.
- Season with salt and pepper to taste.
- Garnish with fresh herbs if desired.
- Serve immediately and enjoy this protein-packed and fiber-rich breakfast!

Health Benefits:

- Whole grain bread provides complex carbohydrates and fiber, promoting satiety and digestive health.
- Avocado is rich in heart-healthy monounsaturated fats and potassium, supporting cardiovascular health and blood pressure regulation.
- Poached egg adds high-quality protein and essential nutrients, including vitamin D and B vitamins, for muscle and nerve function.

Nutritional Value (per serving):

- Calories: 250
- Protein: 13g
- Carbohydrates: 20g
- Fat: 14g

- Fiber: 6g

- Potassium: 300mg

Preparation Time: 10 minutes

5: Sweet Potato Breakfast Hash

Ingredients:

- 1 small sweet potato, peeled and diced

- 1/4 cup diced zucchini

- 1/4 cup diced bell peppers

- 1/4 cup diced onions

- 1 tablespoon olive oil

- 2 large eggs

- Salt and pepper to taste

- Chopped parsley for garnish (optional)

Instructions:

- Heat olive oil in a skillet over medium heat.

- Add diced sweet potatoes to the skillet and cook until tender and slightly crispy, about 8-10 minutes.

- Add diced zucchini, bell peppers, and onions to the skillet and cook until vegetables are tender.

- Create two wells in the hash and crack one egg into each well.

- Cover the skillet and cook until the eggs are cooked to your desired level of doneness, about 3-5 minutes for runny yolks.
- Season with salt and pepper to taste.
- Garnish with chopped parsley if desired and serve hot.
- Enjoy this hearty and nutritious breakfast hash!

Health Benefits:

- Sweet potatoes are a good source of vitamins A and C, potassium, and fiber, supporting heart and digestive health.
- Zucchini and bell peppers add color, flavor, and essential nutrients such as vitamin C and antioxidants.
- Eggs provide high-quality protein and essential amino acids, promoting muscle health and satiety.

Nutritional Value (per serving):

- Calories: 250
- Protein: 10g
- Carbohydrates: 20g
- Fat: 14g
- Fiber: 4g
- Potassium: 350mg

Preparation Time: 20 minutes

6: Greek Yogurt Parfait

Ingredients:

- 1/2 cup low-fat Greek yogurt
- 1/4 cup fresh berries (such as strawberries, blueberries, or raspberries)
- 2 tablespoons chopped almonds or walnuts
- 1 tablespoon unsweetened shredded coconut (optional)
- 1 teaspoon honey (optional)

Instructions:

- In a serving glass or bowl, layer the Greek yogurt, fresh berries, and chopped nuts.
- Repeat the layers until all ingredients are used.
- Drizzle honey on top if desired and sprinkle with shredded coconut for added flavor.
- Serve immediately or refrigerate until ready to eat.
- Enjoy this refreshing and protein-rich breakfast parfait!

Health Benefits:

- Greek yogurt is high in protein and calcium, supporting bone health and muscle function.
- Berries are low in sugar and high in antioxidants, vitamins, and fiber, promoting heart health and immune function.

- Nuts provide heart-healthy fats, protein, and fiber, helping to regulate blood sugar levels and reduce inflammation.

Nutritional Value (per serving):

- Calories: 220
- Protein: 15g
- Carbohydrates: 15g
- Fat: 12g
- Fiber: 4g
- Potassium: 250mg

Preparation Time: 5 minutes

7: Quinoa Breakfast Bowl

Ingredients:

- 1/2 cup cooked quinoa
- 1/4 cup diced apples
- 1 tablespoon chopped almonds or pecans
- 1 tablespoon unsweetened shredded coconut
- 1 teaspoon ground cinnamon
- 1/2 teaspoon vanilla extract
- 1/4 cup unsweetened almond milk

Instructions:

- In a bowl, combine cooked quinoa, diced apples, chopped nuts, shredded coconut, ground cinnamon, and vanilla extract.
- Stir in unsweetened almond milk until well combined.
- Microwave the mixture for 1-2 minutes until warm.
- Stir again and adjust consistency with more almond milk if desired.
- Serve hot and enjoy this nutritious and filling breakfast bowl!

Health Benefits:

- Quinoa is a complete protein source, providing essential amino acids for muscle health and repair.
- Apples are low in potassium and high in fiber, supporting digestive health and blood sugar control.
- Almonds or pecans add heart-healthy fats and protein, helping to promote satiety and regulate blood sugar levels.
- Cinnamon may help improve insulin sensitivity and lower blood sugar levels.

Nutritional Value (per serving):

- Calories: 280
- Protein: 8g

- Carbohydrates: 35g

- Fat: 12g

- Fiber: 6g

- Potassium: 210mg

Preparation Time: 10 minutes

8: Mediterranean Egg Muffins

Ingredients:

- 4 large eggs

- 1/4 cup diced tomatoes

- 1/4 cup chopped spinach

- 2 tablespoons crumbled feta cheese

- 1 tablespoon chopped black olives

- 1 teaspoon olive oil

- Salt and pepper to taste

Instructions:

- Preheat the oven to 350°F (175°C). Grease a muffin tin with olive oil or line with silicone muffin liners.

- In a bowl, whisk the eggs with salt and pepper.

- Divide diced tomatoes, chopped spinach, feta cheese, and black olives evenly among the muffin cups.

- Pour the whisked eggs over the vegetable mixture in each muffin cup, filling about 3/4 full.

- Bake in the preheated oven for 20-25 minutes or until the egg muffins are set and lightly golden on top.

- Remove from the oven and let cool slightly before serving.

- Enjoy these savory Mediterranean egg muffins for a protein-packed breakfast!

Health Benefits:

- Eggs provide high-quality protein and essential nutrients, supporting muscle health and satiety.

- Tomatoes and spinach are rich in vitamins, minerals, and antioxidants, promoting heart health and immune function.

- Feta cheese and olives add Mediterranean flavor and healthy fats, supporting overall health and well-being.

Nutritional Value (per serving - 2 muffins):

- Calories: 220

- Protein: 15g

- Carbohydrates: 4g

- Fat: 15g

- Fiber: 1g

- Potassium: 240mg

Preparation Time: 30 minutes

9: Cottage Cheese Breakfast Bowl

Ingredients:

- 1/2 cup low-fat cottage cheese
- 1/4 cup diced peaches (fresh or canned in juice)
- 1 tablespoon chopped almonds or walnuts
- 1 tablespoon unsweetened shredded coconut
- 1 teaspoon honey (optional)
- 1/4 teaspoon ground cinnamon

Instructions:

- In a bowl, combine low-fat cottage cheese, diced peaches, chopped nuts, shredded coconut, and ground cinnamon.
- Drizzle honey over the mixture if desired.
- Stir until well combined.
- Serve immediately and enjoy this protein-rich and kidney-friendly breakfast bowl!

Health Benefits:

- Cottage cheese is high in protein and low in phosphorus and potassium, making it an excellent choice for individuals with CKD Stage 4.
- Peaches add natural sweetness and are low in potassium, providing vitamins A and C for immune function and skin health.

- Almonds or walnuts offer heart-healthy fats and protein, helping to promote satiety and regulate blood sugar levels.

- Cinnamon may help improve insulin sensitivity and lower blood sugar levels.

Nutritional Value (per serving):

- Calories: 220
- Protein: 15g
- Carbohydrates: 15g
- Fat: 10g
- Fiber: 2g
- Potassium: 200mg

Preparation Time: 5 minutes

10: Avocado Toast with Poached Egg

Ingredients:

- 1 slice whole grain bread, toasted
- 1/2 ripe avocado, mashed
- 1 large egg
- Salt and pepper to taste
- Chopped fresh herbs (such as parsley or chives) for garnish

Instructions:

- Toast the whole grain bread until golden brown.

- Spread the mashed avocado evenly on top of the toast.
- Fill a small saucepan with water and bring it to a gentle simmer over medium heat.
- Crack the egg into a small bowl or ramekin.
- Carefully slide the egg into the simmering water and poach for 3-4 minutes, until the egg white is set but the yolk is still runny.
- Use a slotted spoon to remove the poached egg from the water and place it on top of the avocado toast.
- Season with salt and pepper to taste.
- Garnish with chopped fresh herbs and serve immediately.
- Enjoy this nutritious and satisfying avocado toast with poached egg!

Health Benefits:

- Whole grain bread provides fiber and essential nutrients, supporting digestive health and heart health.
- Avocado is rich in heart-healthy fats and potassium, promoting satiety and cardiovascular health.
- Eggs provide high-quality protein and essential amino acids, supporting muscle health and satiety.

Nutritional Value (per serving):

- Calories: 250

- Protein: 12g

- Carbohydrates: 20g

- Fat: 14g

- Fiber: 8g

- Potassium: 380mg

Preparation Time: 15 minutes

CKD STAGE 4 LUNCH RECIPES FOR SENIORS

1: Salmon Salad with Lemon-Dill Dressing

Ingredients:

- 4 oz cooked salmon, flaked

- 2 cups mixed salad greens

- 1/4 cup sliced cucumbers

- 1/4 cup cherry tomatoes, halved

- 1 tablespoon chopped fresh dill

- 1 tablespoon extra virgin olive oil

- 1 tablespoon lemon juice

- Salt and pepper to taste

Instructions:

- In a large bowl, combine the mixed salad greens, sliced cucumbers, cherry tomatoes, and flaked salmon.

- In a small bowl, whisk together the extra virgin olive oil, lemon juice, chopped fresh dill, salt, and pepper to make the dressing.
- Drizzle the dressing over the salad and toss gently to coat.

Divide the salad into serving bowls and garnish with additional fresh dill if desired.

Serve immediately and enjoy this refreshing and protein-rich salmon salad!

Health Benefits:

- Salmon is a rich source of omega-3 fatty acids, which have anti-inflammatory properties and support heart health.
- Mixed salad greens, cucumbers, and tomatoes provide essential vitamins, minerals, and antioxidants, promoting overall health and well-being.
- Extra virgin olive oil offers heart-healthy fats and antioxidants, helping to reduce inflammation and support cardiovascular health.
- Lemon juice adds flavor and vitamin C without adding excess sodium.

Nutritional Value (per serving):

- Calories: 250
- Protein: 20g

- Carbohydrates: 6g

- Fat: 16g

- Fiber: 2g

- Potassium: 400mg

Preparation Time: 15 minutes

2: Turkey and Avocado Wrap

Ingredients:

- 2 whole grain wraps or tortillas

- 4 oz sliced turkey breast

- 1/2 avocado, sliced

- 1/4 cup shredded lettuce

- 2 tablespoons hummus

- 1 tablespoon chopped fresh cilantro

- Salt and pepper to taste

Instructions:

- Lay out the whole grain wraps or tortillas on a clean surface.

- Spread 1 tablespoon of hummus evenly over each wrap.

- Layer the sliced turkey breast, avocado slices, shredded lettuce, and chopped fresh cilantro on top of the hummus.

- Season with salt and pepper to taste.

- Roll up the wraps tightly, folding in the sides as you go.

- Slice the wraps in half diagonally and serve immediately.

- Enjoy this protein-packed and fiber-rich turkey and avocado wrap!

Health Benefits:

- Turkey breast is a lean source of protein, providing essential amino acids for muscle health and repair.

- Avocado is rich in heart-healthy fats and potassium, promoting satiety and cardiovascular health.

- Whole grain wraps or tortillas offer fiber and essential nutrients, supporting digestive health and blood sugar control.

- Hummus provides plant-based protein and fiber, helping to regulate blood sugar levels and reduce inflammation.

Nutritional Value (per serving):

- Calories: 300

- Protein: 20g

- Carbohydrates: 25g

- Fat: 15g

- Fiber: 8g

- Potassium: 350mg

Preparation Time: 10 minutes

3: Quinoa and Vegetable Stir-Fry

Ingredients:

- 1/2 cup cooked quinoa
- 1/4 cup diced carrots
- 1/4 cup diced bell peppers (any color)
- 1/4 cup sliced mushrooms
- 1/4 cup snap peas
- 2 tablespoons low-sodium soy sauce
- 1 tablespoon olive oil
- 1 clove garlic, minced
- 1 teaspoon grated ginger
- 1 tablespoon chopped green onions (optional)
- Sesame seeds for garnish (optional)

Instructions:

- Heat olive oil in a large skillet or wok over medium heat.
- Add minced garlic and grated ginger to the skillet and cook until fragrant, about 1 minute.
- Add diced carrots, bell peppers, mushrooms, and snap peas to the skillet. Stir-fry until vegetables are tender-crisp, about 5-7 minutes.
- Add cooked quinoa to the skillet and stir to combine with the vegetables.

- Pour low-sodium soy sauce over the quinoa and vegetable mixture. Stir well to coat evenly.
- Cook for an additional 2-3 minutes until everything is heated through.
- Garnish with chopped green onions and sesame seeds if desired.
- Serve hot and enjoy this flavorful and nutrient-rich quinoa and vegetable stir-fry!

Health Benefits:

- Quinoa is a complete protein source, providing essential amino acids for muscle health and repair.
- Carrots, bell peppers, mushrooms, and snap peas offer vitamins, minerals, and antioxidants, supporting immune function and overall health.
- Low-sodium soy sauce adds flavor without adding excess sodium, making it suitable for individuals with CKD Stage 4.
- Olive oil provides heart-healthy fats and anti-inflammatory properties, supporting cardiovascular health.

Nutritional Value (per serving):

- Calories: 280
- Protein: 10g

- Carbohydrates: 40g

- Fat: 8g

- Fiber: 6g

- Potassium: 350mg

Preparation Time: 20 minutes

4: Lentil and Vegetable Soup

Ingredients:

- 1/2 cup dried green or brown lentils, rinsed and drained

- 2 cups low-sodium vegetable broth

- 1/2 cup diced onions

- 1/4 cup diced carrots

- 1/4 cup diced celery

- 1/4 cup diced tomatoes

- 1 clove garlic, minced

- 1 bay leaf

- 1/2 teaspoon dried thyme

- Salt and pepper to taste

- Chopped fresh parsley for garnish (optional)

Instructions: In a large pot, combine rinsed lentils, low-sodium vegetable broth, diced onions, carrots, celery, diced tomatoes, minced garlic, bay leaf, and dried thyme.

- Bring the mixture to a boil over medium-high heat.

- Reduce the heat to low, cover, and simmer for 20-25 minutes or until the lentils and vegetables are tender.

- Season with salt and pepper to taste.

- Remove the bay leaf from the soup and discard.

- Ladle the soup into serving bowls and garnish with chopped fresh parsley if desired.

- Serve hot and enjoy this hearty and nutritious lentil and vegetable soup!

Health Benefits:

- Lentils are high in protein, fiber, and essential nutrients, supporting digestive health and blood sugar control.

- Onions, carrots, celery, tomatoes, and garlic provide vitamins, minerals, and antioxidants, promoting immune function and heart health.

- Vegetable broth adds flavor and depth to the soup without adding excess sodium, making it suitable for individuals with CKD Stage 4.

- Herbs like thyme and parsley offer additional flavor and antioxidant benefits.

Nutritional Value (per serving):

- Calories: 220

- Protein: 12g

- Carbohydrates: 35g

- Fat: 1g

- Fiber: 10g

- Potassium: 450mg

Preparation Time: 30 minutes

5: Grilled Chicken Salad with Balsamic Vinaigrette

Ingredients:

- 4 oz grilled chicken breast, sliced

- 2 cups mixed salad greens

- 1/4 cup sliced cucumbers

- 1/4 cup sliced strawberries

- 1/4 cup crumbled feta cheese

- 2 tablespoons chopped walnuts

- 1 tablespoon extra virgin olive oil

- 1 tablespoon balsamic vinegar

- Salt and pepper to taste

Instructions:

- In a large bowl, combine the mixed salad greens, sliced cucumbers, sliced strawberries, crumbled feta cheese, and chopped walnuts.

- Top the salad with sliced grilled chicken breast.
- In a small bowl, whisk together the extra virgin olive oil, balsamic vinegar, salt, and pepper to make the dressing.
- Drizzle the dressing over the salad and toss gently to coat.
- Divide the salad into serving bowls and serve immediately.
- Enjoy this delicious and protein-rich grilled chicken salad with balsamic vinaigrette!

Health Benefits:

- Grilled chicken breast is a lean source of protein, providing essential amino acids for muscle health and repair.
- Mixed salad greens, cucumbers, strawberries, and walnuts offer vitamins, minerals, and antioxidants, supporting overall health and well-being.
- Feta cheese adds flavor and calcium without adding excess phosphorus, making it suitable for individuals with CKD Stage 4.
- Extra virgin olive oil and balsamic vinegar provide heart-healthy fats and antioxidants, helping to reduce inflammation and support cardiovascular health.

Nutritional Value (per serving):

- Calories: 320
- Protein: 25g

- Carbohydrates: 10g
- Fat: 20g
- Fiber: 3g
- Potassium: 400mg

Preparation Time: 20 minutes

6: Tuna and White Bean Salad

Ingredients:

- 1 can (5 oz) water-packed tuna, drained
- 1 cup cooked white beans (cannellini or navy beans), drained and rinsed
- 1/4 cup diced red onions
- 1/4 cup chopped celery
- 1/4 cup diced red bell peppers
- 1 tablespoon chopped fresh parsley
- 1 tablespoon lemon juice
- 1 tablespoon extra virgin olive oil
- Salt and pepper to taste

Instructions:

- In a large bowl, combine the drained tuna, cooked white beans, diced red onions, chopped celery, diced red bell peppers, and chopped fresh parsley.

- Drizzle the lemon juice and extra virgin olive oil over the salad.
- Season with salt and pepper to taste.
- Toss gently to combine all the ingredients.
- Serve immediately or refrigerate for 30 minutes to allow the flavors to meld.
- Enjoy this protein-packed and fiber-rich tuna and white bean salad!

Health Benefits:

- Water-packed tuna is a lean source of protein and omega-3 fatty acids, supporting heart health and muscle function.
- White beans provide protein, fiber, and essential nutrients, promoting digestive health and blood sugar control.
- Red onions, celery, red bell peppers, and parsley offer vitamins, minerals, and antioxidants, supporting immune function and overall health.
- Lemon juice and extra virgin olive oil add flavor and heart-healthy fats without adding excess sodium.

Nutritional Value (per serving):

- Calories: 280
- Protein: 20g
- Carbohydrates: 20g

- Fat: 12g

- Fiber: 6g

- Potassium: 450mg

Preparation Time: 15 minutes

7: Eggplant and Chickpea Stew

Ingredients:

- 1 small eggplant, diced

- 1 can (15 oz) chickpeas, drained and rinsed

- 1/2 cup diced tomatoes (fresh or canned)

- 1/4 cup diced onions

- 1/4 cup diced carrots

- 1/4 cup diced celery

- 2 cloves garlic, minced

- 1 teaspoon dried oregano

- 1/2 teaspoon paprika

- 2 cups low-sodium vegetable broth

- Salt and pepper to taste

- Chopped fresh parsley for garnish (optional)

Instructions:

- In a large pot, heat a small amount of olive oil over medium heat.

- Add diced onions, carrots, celery, and minced garlic to the pot. Cook until vegetables are softened, about 5 minutes.

- Add diced eggplant to the pot and cook for another 5 minutes, until slightly browned.

- Stir in diced tomatoes, chickpeas, dried oregano, paprika, and low-sodium vegetable broth.

- Bring the stew to a boil, then reduce the heat to low and simmer for 20-25 minutes, until the vegetables are tender and the flavors are well combined.

- Season with salt and pepper to taste.

- Ladle the stew into serving bowls and garnish with chopped fresh parsley if desired.

- Serve hot and enjoy this hearty and nutritious eggplant and chickpea stew!

Health Benefits:

- Eggplant is low in potassium and provides fiber, vitamins, and minerals, supporting digestive health and blood sugar control.

- Chickpeas are rich in protein and fiber, promoting satiety and cardiovascular health.

- Tomatoes offer lycopene, a powerful antioxidant that may help reduce inflammation and protect against chronic diseases.

- Onions, carrots, celery, and garlic provide additional vitamins, minerals, and antioxidants, supporting immune function and overall health.

Nutritional Value (per serving):

- Calories: 250
- Protein: 10g
- Carbohydrates: 40g
- Fat: 5g
- Fiber: 10g
- Potassium: 400mg

Preparation Time: 40 minutes

8: Tofu and Vegetable Stir-Fry

Ingredients:

- 8 oz extra firm tofu, drained and cubed
- 1 cup broccoli florets
- 1/2 cup sliced bell peppers (any color)
- 1/2 cup sliced carrots
- 1/4 cup sliced mushrooms
- 2 tablespoons low-sodium soy sauce
- 1 tablespoon sesame oil
- 1 clove garlic, minced

- 1 teaspoon grated ginger

- 2 green onions, chopped (for garnish)

- Sesame seeds (for garnish, optional)

Instructions:

- In a large skillet or wok, heat sesame oil over medium-high heat.

- Add minced garlic and grated ginger to the skillet and cook until fragrant, about 1 minute.

- Add cubed tofu to the skillet and cook until lightly browned on all sides, about 5-7 minutes.

- Add broccoli florets, sliced bell peppers, sliced carrots, and sliced mushrooms to the skillet. Stir-fry until vegetables are tender-crisp, about 5-7 minutes.

- Pour low-sodium soy sauce over the tofu and vegetable mixture. Stir well to coat evenly.

- Cook for an additional 2-3 minutes until everything is heated through.

- Garnish with chopped green onions and sesame seeds if desired.

- Serve hot and enjoy this protein-packed and nutrient-rich tofu and vegetable stir-fry!

Health Benefits: Tofu is a plant-based source of protein and calcium, supporting muscle health and bone health.

- Broccoli, bell peppers, carrots, and mushrooms offer vitamins, minerals, and antioxidants, promoting immune function and cardiovascular health.

- Low-sodium soy sauce adds flavor without adding excess sodium, making it suitable for individuals with CKD Stage 4.

- Sesame oil provides heart-healthy fats and adds a nutty flavor to the stir-fry.

Nutritional Value (per serving):

- Calories: 280
- Protein: 20g
- Carbohydrates: 15g
- Fat: 15g
- Fiber: 5g
- Potassium: 400mg

Preparation Time: 30 minutes

9: Salmon and Asparagus Quinoa Salad

Ingredients:

- 4 oz grilled or baked salmon fillet, flaked
- 1 cup cooked quinoa
- 1/2 cup chopped asparagus
- 1/4 cup diced red bell peppers

- 1/4 cup cherry tomatoes, halved
- 2 tablespoons chopped fresh parsley
- 1 tablespoon lemon juice
- 1 tablespoon extra-virgin olive oil
- Salt and pepper to taste

Instructions:

- In a large bowl, combine cooked quinoa, chopped asparagus, diced red bell peppers, cherry tomatoes, and chopped fresh parsley.
- Add flaked salmon to the bowl.
- In a small bowl, whisk together lemon juice, extra virgin olive oil, salt, and pepper to make the dressing.
- Drizzle the dressing over the salad and toss gently to combine.
- Divide the salad into serving bowls and serve immediately.
- Enjoy this protein-rich and fiber-packed salmon and asparagus quinoa salad!

Health Benefits:

- Salmon is rich in omega-3 fatty acids, which have anti-inflammatory properties and support heart health.
- Quinoa provides protein, fiber, and essential nutrients, promoting digestive health and blood sugar control.

- Asparagus offers vitamins, minerals, and antioxidants, supporting immune function and overall health.
- Red bell peppers and cherry tomatoes are rich in vitamin C and other antioxidants, helping to reduce inflammation and support cellular health.

Nutritional Value (per serving):

- Calories: 300
- Protein: 25g
- Carbohydrates: 20g
- Fat: 15g
- Fiber: 5g
- Potassium: 450mg

Preparation Time: 30 minutes

10: Turkey and Spinach Wrap

Ingredients:

- 4 oz cooked turkey breast, sliced
- 1 whole wheat or spinach tortilla wrap
- 1/2 cup fresh spinach leaves
- 1/4 cup diced cucumbers
- 1/4 cup diced tomatoes
- 2 tablespoons hummus

- 1 tablespoon Greek yogurt

- 1 teaspoon lemon juice

- Salt and pepper to taste

Instructions:

- Lay the tortilla wrap flat on a clean surface.

- Spread hummus evenly over the tortilla wrap.

- Layer fresh spinach leaves, sliced cooked turkey breast, diced cucumbers, and diced tomatoes on top of the hummus.

- In a small bowl, mix Greek yogurt, lemon juice, salt, and pepper to make the dressing.

- Drizzle the dressing over the filling.

- Roll up the tortilla wrap tightly.

- Slice the wrap in half diagonally.

- Serve immediately or wrap in foil for later.

Health Benefits:

- Turkey breast is a lean source of protein, providing essential amino acids for muscle health and repair.

- Spinach is rich in iron and other vitamins and minerals, supporting energy production and immune function.

- Cucumbers and tomatoes offer hydration and vitamins, promoting overall health and well-being.

- Hummus provides plant-based protein and fiber, promoting satiety and digestive health.

Nutritional Value (per serving):

- Calories: 280
- Protein: 20g
- Carbohydrates: 25g
- Fat: 10g
- Fiber: 5g
- Potassium: 300mg

Preparation Time: 15 minutes

CKD STAGE 4 DINNER RECIPES FOR SENIORS

1. Lemon Herb Baked Cod with Roasted Vegetables

Ingredients:

- 4 oz cod fillet
- 1 lemon, sliced
- 1 tablespoon chopped fresh parsley
- 1 tablespoon chopped fresh dill
- 1 tablespoon olive oil
- Salt and pepper to taste
- 1 cup mixed vegetables (such as carrots, bell peppers, and zucchini), chopped

- Cooking spray

Instructions:

- Preheat the oven to 375°F (190°C).
- Season the cod fillet with salt, pepper, chopped fresh parsley, and chopped fresh dill.
- Place the seasoned cod fillet on a baking sheet lined with parchment paper or aluminum foil.
- Arrange lemon slices on top of the cod fillet.
- Drizzle olive oil over the cod fillet and lemon slices.
- In a separate bowl, toss the mixed vegetables with olive oil, salt, and pepper.
- Spread the mixed vegetables around the cod fillet on the baking sheet.
- Bake in the preheated oven for 15-20 minutes, or until the cod is cooked through and the vegetables are tender.
- Remove from the oven and serve hot.

Health Benefits:

- Cod is a lean source of protein and contains heart-healthy omega-3 fatty acids.
- Mixed vegetables provide essential vitamins, minerals, and dietary fiber, supporting overall health and digestion.

- Lemon adds a burst of flavor and provides vitamin C, which helps boost immunity.

Nutritional Value (per serving):

- Calories: 200
- Protein: 20g
- Carbohydrates: 10g
- Fat: 8g
- Fiber: 4g
- Potassium: 500mg

Preparation Time: 30 minutes

2: Quinoa and Vegetable Stir-Fry

Ingredients:

- 1/2 cup quinoa, rinsed
- 1 cup water or low-sodium vegetable broth
- 1 tablespoon olive oil
- 1/4 cup diced onions
- 1/2 cup sliced bell peppers (any color)
- 1/2 cup sliced carrots
- 1/2 cup sliced mushrooms
- 1/2 cup broccoli florets
- 2 tablespoons low-sodium soy sauce

- 1 teaspoon sesame oil

- 1 teaspoon grated ginger

- 1 clove garlic, minced

- Salt and pepper to taste

- Chopped green onions for garnish (optional)

Instructions:

- In a medium saucepan, combine quinoa and water or vegetable broth. Bring to a boil, then reduce heat to low, cover, and simmer for 15-20 minutes, or until quinoa is cooked and water is absorbed. Remove from heat and let it sit covered for 5 minutes.

- Heat olive oil in a large skillet or wok over medium-high heat. Add diced onions, sliced bell peppers, sliced carrots, sliced mushrooms, and broccoli florets. Stir-fry for 5-7 minutes, or until vegetables are tender-crisp.

- Add minced garlic and grated ginger to the skillet and cook for an additional 1 minute.

- Add cooked quinoa to the skillet and stir to combine with the vegetables.

- Drizzle low-sodium soy sauce and sesame oil over the quinoa and vegetable mixture. Stir well to coat evenly.

- Season with salt and pepper to taste.

- Garnish with chopped green onions if desired.

- Serve hot and enjoy this nutritious and flavorful quinoa and vegetable stir-fry!

Health Benefits:

- Quinoa is a complete protein and contains essential amino acids, making it an excellent plant-based protein source for individuals with CKD Stage 4.
- Mixed vegetables provide vitamins, minerals, and antioxidants, supporting immune function and overall health.
- Garlic and ginger offer anti-inflammatory properties and may help improve circulation and reduce blood pressure.
- Low-sodium soy sauce adds flavor without adding excess sodium, making it suitable for individuals with CKD Stage 4.

Nutritional Value (per serving):

- Calories: 250
- Protein: 10g
- Carbohydrates: 35g
- Fat: 8g
- Fiber: 6g
- Potassium: 300mg

Preparation Time: 30 minutes

Ingredients:

- 4 oz boneless, skinless chicken breast, diced
- 1 cup diced sweet potatoes
- 1 cup diced zucchini
- 1/2 cup diced onions
- 1/2 cup diced bell peppers (any color)
- 1 clove garlic, minced
- 1 tablespoon olive oil
- 1 teaspoon dried thyme
- 1 teaspoon dried rosemary
- Salt and pepper to taste
- Cooking spray

Instructions:

- Preheat the oven to 375°F (190°C). Lightly grease a baking dish with cooking spray.
- In a large bowl, combine diced chicken breast, sweet potatoes, zucchini, onions, bell peppers, minced garlic, olive oil, dried thyme, dried rosemary, salt, and pepper. Toss until everything is evenly coated.
- Transfer the mixture to the prepared baking dish and spread it out into an even layer.

- Cover the baking dish with aluminum foil and bake in the preheated oven for 25-30 minutes.
- Remove the foil and bake for an additional 10-15 minutes, or until the chicken is cooked through and the vegetables are tender.
- Remove from the oven and let it cool for a few minutes before serving.
- Serve hot and enjoy this delicious and nutritious baked chicken and vegetable casserole!

Health Benefits:

- Chicken breast is a lean source of protein and provides essential amino acids for muscle health and repair.
- Sweet potatoes are rich in fiber, vitamins, and minerals, supporting digestive health and blood sugar control.
- Zucchini, onions, and bell peppers offer additional vitamins, minerals, and antioxidants, promoting immune function and overall health.
- Olive oil provides heart-healthy fats and adds flavor to the dish.

Nutritional Value (per serving):

- Calories: 250
- Protein: 25g

- Carbohydrates: 20g

- Fat: 8g

- Fiber: 5g

- Potassium: 400mg

Preparation Time: 45 minutes

4: Lentil and Vegetable Soup

Ingredients:

- 1/2 cup dried lentils, rinsed

- 4 cups low-sodium vegetable broth

- 1 cup diced carrots

- 1 cup diced celery

- 1 cup diced onions

- 1 cup diced tomatoes (fresh or canned)

- 2 cloves garlic, minced

- 1 teaspoon dried thyme

- 1 teaspoon dried rosemary

- Salt and pepper to taste

- Chopped fresh parsley for garnish (optional)

Instructions:

- In a large pot, combine dried lentils and low-sodium vegetable broth. Bring to a boil over medium-high heat.

- Reduce the heat to low, cover, and simmer for 20-25 minutes, or until lentils are tender.
- Add diced carrots, diced celery, diced onions, diced tomatoes, minced garlic, dried thyme, dried rosemary, salt, and pepper to the pot. Stir to combine.
- Continue to simmer for an additional 10-15 minutes, or until the vegetables are tender.
- Adjust seasoning with salt and pepper to taste.
- Ladle the soup into serving bowls and garnish with chopped fresh parsley if desired.
- Serve hot and enjoy this hearty and comforting lentil and vegetable soup!

Health Benefits:

- Lentils are a rich source of plant-based protein and fiber, promoting satiety and digestive health.
- Carrots, celery, onions, and tomatoes provide vitamins, minerals, and antioxidants, supporting immune function and cardiovascular health.
- Garlic, thyme, and rosemary offer anti-inflammatory properties and may help lower blood pressure and cholesterol levels.

Nutritional Value (per serving):

- Calories: 200
- Protein: 15g
- Carbohydrates: 30g
- Fat: 2g
- Fiber: 10g
- Potassium: 500mg

Preparation Time: 60 minutes

5: Eggplant and Chickpea Curry

Ingredients:

- 1 large eggplant, diced
- 1 can (15 oz) chickpeas, drained and rinsed
- 1 cup diced onions
- 2 cloves garlic, minced
- 1 tablespoon olive oil
- 1 can (14 oz) diced tomatoes (low-sodium)
- 1 can (14 oz) coconut milk (light)
- 2 teaspoons curry powder
- 1 teaspoon ground cumin
- 1 teaspoon ground turmeric
- Salt and pepper to taste
- Chopped fresh cilantro for garnish (optional)

- Cooked brown rice for serving

Instructions:

- Heat olive oil in a large skillet over medium heat. Add diced onions and minced garlic. Sauté until onions are translucent and garlic is fragrant, about 2-3 minutes.
- Add diced eggplant to the skillet and cook until slightly softened, about 5-7 minutes.
- Stir in curry powder, ground cumin, and ground turmeric. Cook for an additional 1-2 minutes until fragrant.
- Add diced tomatoes (with their juices), chickpeas, and coconut milk to the skillet. Stir to combine.
- Bring the mixture to a simmer and let it cook for 15-20 minutes, stirring occasionally, until the eggplant is tender and the flavors are well combined.
- Season with salt and pepper to taste.
- Serve the eggplant and chickpea curry hot over cooked brown rice.
- Garnish with chopped fresh cilantro if desired.
- Enjoy this flavorful and nutritious eggplant and chickpea curry!

Health Benefits:

- Eggplant is low in potassium and phosphorus, making it suitable for individuals with CKD Stage 4. It provides fiber, antioxidants, and vitamins.
- Chickpeas are a good source of plant-based protein and fiber, promoting satiety and digestive health.
- Coconut milk adds creaminess to the curry and provides healthy fats. Opt for light coconut milk to reduce the fat content.

Nutritional Value (per serving, curry only):

- Calories: 250
- Protein: 8g
- Carbohydrates: 30g
- Fat: 12g
- Fiber: 8g
- Potassium: 300mg

Preparation Time: 40 minutes

6: Turkey Meatballs with Zucchini Noodles

Ingredients:

- 4 oz ground turkey breast
- 1/4 cup breadcrumbs (whole wheat or gluten-free)

- 1 egg
- 1/4 cup grated Parmesan cheese
- 1 clove garlic, minced
- 1 teaspoon dried oregano
- 1/2 teaspoon dried basil
- Salt and pepper to taste
- 2 medium zucchinis
- 1 tablespoon olive oil
- 1 can (14 oz) low-sodium tomato sauce
- Chopped fresh parsley for garnish (optional)

Instructions:

- In a large bowl, combine ground turkey breast, breadcrumbs, egg, grated Parmesan cheese, minced garlic, dried oregano, dried basil, salt, and pepper. Mix until well combined.
- Shape the mixture into small meatballs, about 1 inch in diameter.
- Heat olive oil in a large skillet over medium heat. Add the turkey meatballs to the skillet and cook until browned on all sides and cooked through, about 8-10 minutes.
- Spiralize the zucchinis to make zucchini noodles.
- Once the turkey meatballs are cooked, add the low-sodium tomato sauce to the skillet. Stir to coat the meatballs evenly.

- Add the zucchini noodles to the skillet and gently toss with the tomato sauce and meatballs. Cook for 2-3 minutes until the zucchini noodles are tender.

- Remove from heat and garnish with chopped fresh parsley if desired.

- Serve the turkey meatballs and zucchini noodles hot.

- Enjoy this lighter and healthier twist on traditional spaghetti and meatballs!

Health Benefits:

- Ground turkey breast is a lean source of protein and provides essential amino acids for muscle health and repair.

- Zucchini noodles are low in carbohydrates and calories, making them a nutritious alternative to traditional pasta. They provide vitamins, minerals, and antioxidants.

- Tomato sauce adds flavor to the dish and provides lycopene, a powerful antioxidant that may help reduce the risk of chronic diseases.

Nutritional Value (per serving, meatballs and zucchini noodles):

- Calories: 220

- Protein: 20g

- Carbohydrates: 15g

- Fat: 8g

- Fiber: 4g

- Potassium: 400mg

Preparation Time: 30 minutes

7: Salmon and Asparagus Foil Packets

Ingredients:

- 4 oz salmon fillet

- 1/2 cup asparagus spears, trimmed

- 1/4 cup diced red bell pepper

- 1/4 cup diced yellow bell pepper

- 1/4 cup diced red onion

- 1 tablespoon olive oil

- 1 tablespoon lemon juice

- 1 teaspoon dried dill

- Salt and pepper to taste

- Cooking spray

Instructions:

- Preheat the oven to 375°F (190°C). Tear off two large pieces of aluminum foil and lightly coat each with cooking spray.

- Place the salmon fillet in the center of each piece of foil. Arrange the asparagus spears, diced red bell pepper, diced yellow bell pepper, and diced red onion around the salmon.

- Drizzle olive oil and lemon juice over the salmon and vegetables. Sprinkle dried dill, salt, and pepper evenly over each packet.
- Fold the edges of the foil over the salmon and vegetables to create a sealed packet.
- Place the foil packets on a baking sheet and bake in the preheated oven for 15-20 minutes, or until the salmon is cooked through and the vegetables are tender.
- Carefully open the foil packets, being mindful of the steam, and transfer the contents to serving plates.
- Serve hot and enjoy this delicious and nutritious salmon and asparagus foil packets!

Health Benefits:

- Salmon is rich in omega-3 fatty acids, which have anti-inflammatory properties and may help improve heart health.
- Asparagus is low in potassium and provides vitamins A, C, and K, as well as fiber, promoting digestive health and immune function.
- Bell peppers and onions add color and flavor to the dish while providing vitamins, minerals, and antioxidants.

Nutritional Value (per serving):

- Calories: 250

- Protein: 20g

- Carbohydrates: 10g

- Fat: 15g

- Fiber: 3g

- Potassium: 300mg

Preparation Time: 25 minutes

8: Vegetable and Tofu Stir-Fry

Ingredients:

- 4 oz firm tofu, cubed

- 1 cup sliced mushrooms

- 1 cup sliced bell peppers (any color)

- 1 cup sliced zucchini

- 1 cup sliced yellow squash

- 1/4 cup low-sodium soy sauce

- 1 tablespoon sesame oil

- 1 tablespoon cornstarch

- 1 teaspoon grated ginger

- 2 cloves garlic, minced

- 2 green onions, chopped

- Cooked brown rice for serving

Instructions:

- In a small bowl, whisk together low-sodium soy sauce, sesame oil, cornstarch, grated ginger, minced garlic, and chopped green onions to make the sauce. Set aside.
- Heat a non-stick skillet or wok over medium-high heat. Add the cubed tofu and cook until golden brown on all sides, about 5-7 minutes. Remove from the skillet and set aside.
- In the same skillet, add sliced mushrooms, sliced bell peppers, sliced zucchini, and sliced yellow squash. Stir-fry for 5-7 minutes, or until the vegetables are tender-crisp.
- Return the cooked tofu to the skillet and pour the sauce over the tofu and vegetables. Stir to coat evenly.
- Continue to cook for an additional 2-3 minutes, or until the sauce has thickened and everything is heated through.
- Remove from heat and serve the vegetable and tofu stir-fry hot over cooked brown rice.
- Enjoy this flavorful and nutritious vegetable and tofu stir-fry!

Health Benefits:

- Tofu is a plant-based source of protein and provides essential amino acids, promoting muscle health and repair.
- Mushrooms, bell peppers, zucchini, and yellow squash are low in potassium and provide vitamins, minerals, and

antioxidants, supporting immune function and overall health.

- The sauce adds flavor to the dish and is low in sodium, making it suitable for individuals with CKD Stage 4.

Nutritional Value (per serving):

- Calories: 220
- Protein: 15g
- Carbohydrates: 20g
- Fat: 10g
- Fiber: 5g
- Potassium: 350mg

Preparation Time: 30 minutes

9: Quinoa and Black Bean Stuffed Bell Peppers

Ingredients:

- 2 large bell peppers (any color)
- 1/2 cup quinoa, rinsed
- 1 can (15 oz) black beans, drained and rinsed
- 1/2 cup diced tomatoes (fresh or canned)
- 1/4 cup diced onions
- 1/4 cup diced green chilies (optional)
- 1 teaspoon chili powder

- 1/2 teaspoon ground cumin

- Salt and pepper to taste

- 1/4 cup shredded low-fat cheese (optional)

- Chopped fresh cilantro for garnish (optional)

Instructions:

- Preheat the oven to 375°F (190°C). Cut the bell peppers in half lengthwise and remove the seeds and membranes.

- In a medium saucepan, bring 1 cup of water to a boil. Add rinsed quinoa, reduce heat to low, cover, and simmer for 15-20 minutes, or until quinoa is cooked and water is absorbed.

- In a large bowl, combine cooked quinoa, black beans, diced tomatoes, diced onions, diced green chilies (if using), chili powder, ground cumin, salt, and pepper. Mix well to combine.

- Stuff each bell pepper half with the quinoa and black bean mixture, pressing gently to pack it in.

- Place the stuffed bell peppers in a baking dish, cut-side up. If desired, sprinkle shredded low-fat cheese on top of each stuffed pepper.

- Cover the baking dish with aluminum foil and bake in the preheated oven for 25-30 minutes, or until the bell peppers are tender.

- Remove from the oven and let the stuffed bell peppers cool for a few minutes before serving.
- Garnish with chopped fresh cilantro if desired.
- Serve hot and enjoy these delicious and nutritious quinoa and black bean stuffed bell peppers!

Health Benefits:

- Quinoa is a gluten-free whole grain that provides protein, fiber, and essential nutrients, supporting digestive health and blood sugar control.
- Black beans are a good source of plant-based protein and fiber, promoting satiety and digestive health.
- Bell peppers are low in potassium and provide vitamins A, C, and K, as well as antioxidants, supporting immune function and overall health.

Nutritional Value (per serving, one stuffed bell pepper half without cheese):

- Calories: 200
- Protein: 10g
- Carbohydrates: 35g
- Fat: 2g
- Fiber: 8g
- Potassium: 250mg

Preparation Time: 45 minutes

10: Baked Cod with Lemon Herb Sauce

Ingredients:

- 4 oz cod fillet
- 1 tablespoon olive oil
- 1 tablespoon lemon juice
- 1 teaspoon dried dill
- 1 teaspoon dried parsley
- 1/2 teaspoon garlic powder
- Salt and pepper to taste
- Cooking spray
- Lemon wedges for serving

Instructions:

- Preheat the oven to 375°F (190°C). Lightly coat a baking dish with cooking spray.
- Place the cod fillet in the prepared baking dish.
- In a small bowl, whisk together olive oil, lemon juice, dried dill, dried parsley, garlic powder, salt, and pepper to make the sauce.
- Pour the sauce over the cod fillet, spreading it evenly to coat.
- Bake in the preheated oven for 15-20 minutes, or until the cod is opaque and flakes easily with a fork.

- Remove from the oven and let the baked cod cool for a few minutes before serving.
- Serve hot with lemon wedges on the side.
- Enjoy this light and flavorful baked cod with lemon herb sauce!

Health Benefits:

- Cod is a lean source of protein and provides omega-3 fatty acids, which have anti-inflammatory properties and may help improve heart health.
- Olive oil and lemon juice add flavor to the dish and provide heart-healthy fats and antioxidants.

Nutritional Value (per serving):

- Calories: 180
- Protein: 20g
- Carbohydrates: 2g
- Fat: 10g
- Fiber: 0g
- Potassium: 250mg

Preparation Time: 25 minutes

CKD STAGE 4 SNACK RECIPES FOR SENIORS

1: Cottage Cheese and Fruit Bowl

Ingredients:

- 1/2 cup low-fat cottage cheese
- 1/2 cup diced fresh fruit (such as berries, peaches, or melon)
- 1 tablespoon chopped nuts (such as almonds or walnuts)
- 1 teaspoon honey (optional)
- Fresh mint leaves for garnish (optional)

Instructions:

- In a small bowl, scoop the low-fat cottage cheese.
- Top the cottage cheese with diced fresh fruit.
- Sprinkle chopped nuts over the fruit.
- Drizzle honey over the top if desired.
- Garnish with fresh mint leaves for extra freshness and flavor.
- Serve immediately and enjoy this refreshing and protein-rich snack!

Health Benefits:

- Low-fat cottage cheese is a good source of protein and provides essential amino acids for muscle health and repair.

- Fresh fruit adds natural sweetness and provides vitamins, minerals, and antioxidants, supporting overall health and immune function.
- Nuts are rich in heart-healthy fats, fiber, and protein, promoting satiety and cardiovascular health.

Nutritional Value (per serving):

- Calories: 150
- Protein: 12g
- Carbohydrates: 15g
- Fat: 6g
- Fiber: 3g
- Potassium: 200mg

Preparation Time: 5 minutes

2: Veggie Sticks with Hummus

Ingredients:

- 1/2 cup sliced cucumber
- 1/2 cup sliced bell peppers (any color)
- 1/2 cup baby carrots
- 1/4 cup cherry tomatoes
- 1/4 cup hummus (low-sodium)
- Fresh parsley for garnish (optional)

Instructions:

- Wash and prepare the vegetables by slicing the cucumber, bell peppers, and cherry tomatoes into sticks.
- Arrange the sliced vegetables on a plate or serving platter.
- Place the hummus in a small bowl in the center of the plate.
- Garnish with fresh parsley for extra flavor and presentation.
- Serve immediately and enjoy this crunchy and nutritious snack!

Health Benefits:

- Cucumbers, bell peppers, carrots, and cherry tomatoes are low in potassium and provide vitamins, minerals, and antioxidants, promoting immune function and overall health.
- Hummus is a plant-based dip made from chickpeas, tahini, olive oil, lemon juice, and garlic. It provides protein, fiber, and healthy fats, promoting satiety and heart health.

Nutritional Value (per serving):

- Calories: 120
- Protein: 5g
- Carbohydrates: 15g
- Fat: 6g
- Fiber: 5g
- Potassium: 250mg

Preparation Time: 10 minutes

3: Greek Yogurt Parfait

Ingredients:

- 1/2 cup plain Greek yogurt (low-fat)
- 1/4 cup sliced strawberries
- 1/4 cup blueberries
- 1 tablespoon chopped nuts (such as almonds or walnuts)
- 1 teaspoon honey (optional)
- 1 teaspoon ground flaxseed (optional)

Instructions:

- In a serving glass or bowl, layer plain Greek yogurt, sliced strawberries, and blueberries.
- Sprinkle chopped nuts and ground flaxseed over the fruit.
- Drizzle honey over the top if desired.
- Repeat the layering process until all ingredients are used, ending with a layer of fruit on top.
- Serve immediately and enjoy this creamy and nutritious yogurt parfait!

Health Benefits:

- Greek yogurt is high in protein and provides probiotics, promoting gut health and digestive function.

- Strawberries and blueberries are low in potassium and provide vitamins, minerals, and antioxidants, supporting immune function and heart health.

- Nuts and ground flaxseed add crunch and provide heart-healthy fats, fiber, and omega-3 fatty acids, promoting satiety and cardiovascular health.

Nutritional Value (per serving):

- Calories: 180

- Protein: 15g

- Carbohydrates: 20g

- Fat: 6g

- Fiber: 4g

- Potassium: 200mg

Preparation Time: 5 minutes

4: Avocado and Tomato Toast

Ingredients:

- 1 slice whole grain bread (low-sodium)

- 1/4 ripe avocado, mashed

- 1/4 cup cherry tomatoes, sliced

- 1 teaspoon olive oil

- Pinch of sea salt

- Pinch of black pepper

- Fresh basil leaves for garnish (optional)

Instructions:

- Toast the whole grain bread until golden brown and crispy.
- Spread the mashed avocado evenly on top of the toasted bread.
- Arrange sliced cherry tomatoes on top of the mashed avocado.
- Drizzle olive oil over the tomatoes.
- Season with a pinch of sea salt and black pepper to taste.
- Garnish with fresh basil leaves for extra flavor and presentation.
- Serve immediately and enjoy this simple and delicious avocado and tomato toast!

Health Benefits:

- Whole grain bread provides fiber and complex carbohydrates, promoting digestive health and steady energy levels.
- Avocado is rich in heart-healthy fats, fiber, and potassium, promoting satiety and cardiovascular health.
- Cherry tomatoes add freshness and provide vitamins, minerals, and antioxidants, supporting immune function and overall health.

Nutritional Value (per serving):

- Calories: 150
- Protein: 4g
- Carbohydrates: 15g
- Fat: 9g
- Fiber: 5g
- Potassium: 200mg

Preparation Time: 10 minutes

5: Tuna Salad Cucumber Bites

Ingredients:

- 1 cucumber, cut into thick slices
- 1 can (5 oz) tuna, drained
- 2 tablespoons plain Greek yogurt (low-fat)
- 1 tablespoon diced celery
- 1 tablespoon diced red onion
- 1 teaspoon lemon juice
- Salt and pepper to taste
- Fresh parsley for garnish (optional)

Instructions: In a small bowl, mix together drained tuna, plain Greek yogurt, diced celery, diced red onion, and lemon juice until well combined.

- Season the tuna salad with salt and pepper to taste.

- Spoon a small amount of tuna salad onto each cucumber slice.

- Garnish with fresh parsley if desired.

- Serve immediately and enjoy these refreshing and protein-rich tuna salad cucumber bites!

Health Benefits:

- Cucumbers are low in potassium and provide hydration and a crunchy texture, promoting digestive health and hydration.

- Tuna is a lean source of protein and provides omega-3 fatty acids, promoting muscle health and heart health.

- Greek yogurt adds creaminess and provides probiotics, promoting gut health and immune function.

Nutritional Value (per serving):

- Calories: 120

- Protein: 15g

- Carbohydrates: 5g

- Fat: 4g

- Fiber: 1g

- Potassium: 150mg

Preparation Time: 15 minutes

6: Rice Cake with Almond Butter and Banana

Ingredients:

- 1 rice cake (low-sodium)
- 1 tablespoon almond butter (unsweetened)
- 1/2 ripe banana, sliced
- 1 teaspoon honey (optional)
- Pinch of cinnamon (optional)

Instructions:

- Spread almond butter evenly on top of the rice cake.
- Arrange sliced banana on top of the almond butter.
- Drizzle honey over the banana slices if desired.
- Sprinkle a pinch of cinnamon over the top for extra flavor.
- Serve immediately and enjoy this simple and satisfying rice cake with almond butter and banana!

Health Benefits:

- Rice cakes are low in potassium and provide a crunchy base for toppings, promoting satiety and providing energy.
- Almond butter is a source of heart-healthy fats, protein, and fiber, promoting satiety and cardiovascular health.
- Bananas add natural sweetness and provide vitamins, minerals, and fiber, supporting digestive health and immune function.

Nutritional Value (per serving):

- Calories: 150
- Protein: 4g
- Carbohydrates: 20g
- Fat: 7g
- Fiber: 3g
- Potassium: 200mg

Preparation Time: 5 minutes

7: Quinoa Salad Stuffed Bell Peppers

Ingredients:

- 2 large bell peppers (any color), halved and seeds removed
- 1/2 cup cooked quinoa
- 1/4 cup diced cucumber
- 1/4 cup diced tomatoes
- 1/4 cup diced red onion
- 2 tablespoons chopped fresh parsley
- 1 tablespoon lemon juice
- 1 tablespoon olive oil
- Salt and pepper to taste
- Fresh basil leaves for garnish (optional)

Instructions:

- Preheat the oven to 375°F (190°C).
- In a mixing bowl, combine cooked quinoa, diced cucumber, diced tomatoes, diced red onion, chopped fresh parsley, lemon juice, olive oil, salt, and pepper. Mix well.
- Stuff each bell pepper half with the quinoa salad mixture.
- Place the stuffed bell peppers on a baking sheet lined with parchment paper.
- Bake in the preheated oven for 20-25 minutes, or until the bell peppers are tender.
- Remove from the oven and let cool slightly.
- Garnish with fresh basil leaves if desired.
- Serve warm or at room temperature as a nutritious and satisfying snack!

Health Benefits:

- Bell peppers are low in potassium and provide vitamins A and C, antioxidants that support immune function and skin health.
- Quinoa is a gluten-free whole grain and a good source of protein, fiber, and essential amino acids, promoting satiety and digestive health.

- Cucumbers, tomatoes, and red onions add freshness and provide vitamins, minerals, and hydration, supporting overall health.

Nutritional Value (per serving, 1 stuffed bell pepper half):

- Calories: 150
- Protein: 4g
- Carbohydrates: 20g
- Fat: 6g
- Fiber: 4g
- Potassium: 200mg

Preparation Time: 30 minutes

8: Coconut Chia Pudding

Ingredients:

- 1/4 cup chia seeds
- 1 cup unsweetened coconut milk
- 1 tablespoon maple syrup or honey (optional)
- 1/4 teaspoon vanilla extract
- 1/4 cup fresh mixed berries (such as strawberries, blueberries, and raspberries)
- 1 tablespoon unsweetened shredded coconut flakes

Instructions:

- In a mixing bowl, combine chia seeds, coconut milk, maple syrup or honey (if using), and vanilla extract. Stir well to combine.
- Cover the bowl and refrigerate for at least 2 hours or overnight, allowing the chia seeds to absorb the liquid and form a pudding-like consistency.
- Once the chia pudding is set, give it a stir to loosen it up.
- Divide the chia pudding into serving bowls or glasses.
- Top with fresh mixed berries and unsweetened shredded coconut flakes.
- Serve chilled and enjoy this creamy and nutritious coconut chia pudding!

Health Benefits:

- Chia seeds are rich in omega-3 fatty acids, fiber, and protein, promoting satiety and digestive health.
- Coconut milk adds creaminess and provides medium-chain triglycerides (MCTs), a type of fat that may benefit heart health and cognitive function.
- Fresh mixed berries are low in potassium and provide vitamins, minerals, and antioxidants, supporting immune function and overall health.

Nutritional Value (per serving):

- Calories: 180
- Protein: 4g
- Carbohydrates: 15g
- Fat: 10g
- Fiber: 7g
- Potassium: 150mg

Preparation Time: 5 minutes (plus chilling time)

9: Baked Apple Chips

Ingredients:

- 2 medium apples (any variety)
- 1 teaspoon cinnamon
- 1/2 teaspoon granulated sugar (optional)
- Cooking spray or olive oil spray

Instructions:

- Preheat the oven to 200°F (95°C) and line a baking sheet with parchment paper.
- Wash and thinly slice the apples using a mandoline slicer or a sharp knife.
- Arrange the apple slices on the prepared baking sheet in a single layer, ensuring they do not overlap.

- Sprinkle cinnamon evenly over the apple slices. If desired, lightly sprinkle granulated sugar over the top.
- Lightly spray the apple slices with cooking spray or olive oil spray to help them crisp up in the oven.
- Bake in the preheated oven for 1.5 to 2 hours, flipping the apple slices halfway through, until they are crisp and lightly golden brown.
- Remove from the oven and let the apple chips cool completely before serving.
- Enjoy these crispy and naturally sweet baked apple chips as a wholesome snack!

Health Benefits:

- Apples are low in potassium and provide fiber, vitamins, and antioxidants, supporting digestive health and immune function.
- Cinnamon adds warmth and flavor and may help regulate blood sugar levels, promoting overall health and well-being.

Nutritional Value (per serving):

- Calories: 80
- Protein: 0g
- Carbohydrates: 22g
- Fat: 0g

- Fiber: 4g

- Potassium: 100mg

Preparation Time: 10 minutes (plus baking time)

10: Edamame Hummus with Veggie Sticks

Ingredients:

- 1 cup shelled edamame (thawed if using frozen)
- 2 tablespoons tahini
- 1 tablespoon lemon juice
- 1 garlic clove, minced
- 1/2 teaspoon ground cumin
- Salt and pepper to taste
- 2 tablespoons water (or more as needed)
- Assorted vegetable sticks (such as carrot sticks, cucumber slices, and bell pepper strips)

Instructions:

- In a food processor, combine the shelled edamame, tahini, lemon juice, minced garlic, ground cumin, salt, and pepper.
- Process until smooth, scraping down the sides of the bowl as needed.
- With the food processor running, gradually add water, 1 tablespoon at a time, until the hummus reaches your desired consistency.

- Transfer the edamame hummus to a serving bowl.

- Arrange the assorted vegetable sticks around the hummus bowl for dipping.

- Serve immediately and enjoy this protein-rich and nutritious edamame hummus with crunchy vegetable sticks!

Health Benefits:

- Edamame is a good source of plant-based protein, fiber, and essential nutrients, promoting muscle health and satiety.

- Tahini adds creaminess and provides healthy fats and minerals, supporting heart health and cognitive function.

- Assorted vegetable sticks provide vitamins, minerals, and antioxidants, promoting overall health and well-being.

Nutritional Value (per serving, 2 tablespoons of hummus with vegetable sticks):

- Calories: 90

- Protein: 5g

- Carbohydrates: 7g

- Fat: 5g

- Fiber: 3g

- Potassium: 150mg

Preparation Time: 10 minutes

CKD STAGE 4 DESSERT RECIPES FOR SENIORS

1: Berry Yogurt Parfait

Ingredients:

- 1/2 cup plain Greek yogurt (low-fat)
- 1/4 cup mixed berries (such as strawberries, blueberries, and raspberries)
- 1 tablespoon unsweetened shredded coconut flakes
- 1 tablespoon chopped nuts (such as almonds or walnuts)
- 1 teaspoon honey (optional)

Instructions:

- In a serving glass or bowl, layer plain Greek yogurt, mixed berries, unsweetened shredded coconut flakes, and chopped nuts.
- Repeat the layers until all ingredients are used, ending with a layer of berries on top.
- Drizzle honey over the top if desired for added sweetness.
- Serve immediately and enjoy this refreshing and nutritious berry yogurt parfait!

Health Benefits:

- Greek yogurt is a good source of protein and calcium, promoting muscle health and bone health.

- Mixed berries are low in potassium and provide vitamins, minerals, and antioxidants, supporting immune function and heart health.

- Coconut flakes and chopped nuts add texture and provide healthy fats and fiber, promoting satiety and digestive health.

Nutritional Value (per serving):

- Calories: 150
- Protein: 10g
- Carbohydrates: 15g
- Fat: 6g
- Fiber: 4g
- Potassium: 200mg

Preparation Time: 5 minutes

2: Baked Cinnamon Apples

Ingredients:

- 2 medium apples (any variety), cored and sliced
- 1 tablespoon unsalted butter, melted
- 1 tablespoon maple syrup or honey
- 1/2 teaspoon ground cinnamon
- 1/4 teaspoon ground nutmeg
- 1/4 teaspoon vanilla extract

- 2 tablespoons chopped nuts (such as pecans or walnuts), optional

Instructions:

- Preheat the oven to 375°F (190°C) and line a baking sheet with parchment paper.
- In a mixing bowl, combine sliced apples, melted unsalted butter, maple syrup or honey, ground cinnamon, ground nutmeg, and vanilla extract. Toss until the apples are evenly coated.
- Spread the apple slices in a single layer on the prepared baking sheet.
- Bake in the preheated oven for 20-25 minutes, or until the apples are tender and lightly caramelized, stirring halfway through.
- Remove from the oven and let the baked cinnamon apples cool slightly.
- Serve warm, sprinkled with chopped nuts if desired.
- Enjoy these delicious and comforting baked cinnamon apples as a satisfying dessert!

Health Benefits: Apples are low in potassium and provide fiber, vitamins, and antioxidants, supporting digestive health and immune function.

- Cinnamon adds warmth and flavor and may help regulate blood sugar levels, promoting overall health and well-being.
- Nuts provide healthy fats, protein, and fiber, promoting heart health and satiety.

Nutritional Value (per serving):

- Calories: 150
- Protein: 2g
- Carbohydrates: 25g
- Fat: 6g
- Fiber: 5g
- Potassium: 150mg

Preparation Time: 30 minutes

3: Chia Seed Pudding with Mango

Ingredients:

- 1/4 cup chia seeds
- 1 cup unsweetened almond milk
- 1 tablespoon maple syrup or honey
- 1/2 teaspoon vanilla extract
- 1 ripe mango, diced
- 1 tablespoon unsweetened shredded coconut flakes

Instructions:

- In a mixing bowl, combine chia seeds, unsweetened almond milk, maple syrup or honey, and vanilla extract. Stir well to combine.
- Cover the bowl and refrigerate for at least 2 hours or overnight, allowing the chia seeds to absorb the liquid and form a pudding-like consistency.
- Once the chia pudding is set, give it a stir to loosen it up.
- Divide the chia pudding into serving bowls or glasses.
- Top with diced mango and unsweetened shredded coconut flakes.
- Serve chilled and enjoy this creamy and tropical chia seed pudding with mango!

Health Benefits:

- Chia seeds are rich in omega-3 fatty acids, fiber, and protein, promoting satiety and digestive health.
- Almond milk is low in potassium and provides vitamins and minerals, supporting bone health and heart health.
- Mango is low in potassium and provides vitamins, minerals, and antioxidants, supporting immune function and eye health.

Nutritional Value (per serving):

- Calories: 150
- Protein: 4g
- Carbohydrates: 20g
- Fat: 6g
- Fiber: 7g
- Potassium: 200mg

Preparation Time: 5 minutes (plus chilling time)

4: Baked Pear with Honey and Cinnamon

Ingredients:

- 2 ripe pears, halved and cored
- 1 tablespoon unsalted butter, melted
- 1 tablespoon honey
- 1/2 teaspoon ground cinnamon
- 1/4 teaspoon ground nutmeg
- 2 tablespoons chopped walnuts (optional)

Instructions:

- Preheat the oven to 375°F (190°C) and line a baking sheet with parchment paper.
- Place the pear halves, cut side up, on the prepared baking sheet.

- In a small bowl, combine melted unsalted butter, honey, ground cinnamon, and ground nutmeg. Mix well.
- Brush the honey mixture over the pear halves, coating them evenly.
- Bake in the preheated oven for 20-25 minutes, or until the pears are tender and lightly caramelized.
- Remove from the oven and let the baked pears cool slightly.
- Serve warm, sprinkled with chopped walnuts if desired.
- Enjoy these comforting and naturally sweet baked pears as a delightful dessert!

Health Benefits:

- Pears are low in potassium and provide fiber, vitamins, and antioxidants, supporting digestive health and heart health.
- Honey adds natural sweetness and provides antioxidants and antimicrobial properties, promoting overall health and well-being.
- Cinnamon and nutmeg add warmth and flavor and may help regulate blood sugar levels, supporting metabolic health.

Nutritional Value (per serving):

- Calories: 150
- Protein: 2g
- Carbohydrates: 30g

- Fat: 4g

- Fiber: 6g

- Potassium: 150mg

Preparation Time: 30 minutes

5: Coconut Chia Popsicles

Ingredients:

- 1/4 cup chia seeds

- 1 cup unsweetened coconut milk

- 1 tablespoon honey or maple syrup

- 1/2 teaspoon vanilla extract

- 1/4 cup unsweetened shredded coconut flakes

Instructions:

- In a mixing bowl, combine chia seeds, coconut milk, honey or maple syrup, and vanilla extract. Stir well to combine.

- Cover the bowl and refrigerate for at least 2 hours or overnight, allowing the chia seeds to absorb the liquid and form a pudding-like consistency.

- Once the chia pudding is set, stir in the unsweetened shredded coconut flakes.

- Pour the mixture into popsicle molds, leaving a little space at the top for expansion.

- Insert popsicle sticks into each mold and freeze for at least 4 hours, or until the popsicles are completely frozen.
- Remove the popsicles from the molds and serve immediately.
- Enjoy these creamy and tropical coconut chia popsicles as a refreshing dessert or snack!

Health Benefits:

- Chia seeds are rich in omega-3 fatty acids, fiber, and protein, promoting satiety and digestive health.
- Coconut milk provides healthy fats and minerals, supporting heart health and immune function.
- Honey or maple syrup adds natural sweetness and provides antioxidants and antimicrobial properties, promoting overall health and well-being.

Nutritional Value (per serving):

- Calories: 120
- Protein: 2g
- Carbohydrates: 10g
- Fat: 8g
- Fiber: 4g
- Potassium: 100mg

Preparation Time: 5 minutes (plus chilling time)

6: Baked Banana with Almond Butter

Ingredients:

- 2 ripe bananas, peeled and halved lengthwise
- 2 tablespoons almond butter
- 1 tablespoon unsweetened shredded coconut flakes
- 1 tablespoon chopped almonds

Instructions:

- Preheat the oven to 375°F (190°C) and line a baking sheet with parchment paper.
- Place the banana halves, cut side up, on the prepared baking sheet.
- Spread almond butter evenly over each banana half.
- Sprinkle unsweetened shredded coconut flakes and chopped almonds over the almond butter.
- Bake in the preheated oven for 10-12 minutes, or until the bananas are tender and lightly golden brown.
- Remove from the oven and let the baked bananas cool slightly.
- Serve warm, sprinkled with additional coconut flakes and almonds if desired.
- Enjoy these indulgent and wholesome baked bananas with almond butter as a satisfying dessert!

Health Benefits:

- Bananas are low in potassium and provide fiber, vitamins, and minerals, supporting digestive health and heart health.
- Almond butter provides healthy fats, protein, and fiber, promoting satiety and supporting brain health.
- Coconut flakes and chopped almonds add texture and provide additional nutrients, such as vitamins, minerals, and antioxidants.

Nutritional Value (per serving):

- Calories: 200
- Protein: 4g
- Carbohydrates: 25g
- Fat: 10g
- Fiber: 6g
- Potassium: 200mg

Preparation Time: 15 minutes

7: Baked Apple Slices with Cinnamon

Ingredients:

- 2 medium apples, cored and sliced
- 1 tablespoon unsalted butter, melted
- 1 teaspoon ground cinnamon

- 1 tablespoon chopped pecans or walnuts (optional)
- 1 tablespoon honey (optional)

Instructions:

- Preheat the oven to 375°F (190°C) and line a baking sheet with parchment paper.
- In a mixing bowl, toss the apple slices with melted unsalted butter and ground cinnamon until evenly coated.
- Spread the apple slices in a single layer on the prepared baking sheet.
- Bake in the preheated oven for 20-25 minutes, or until the apples are tender and lightly caramelized.
- Remove from the oven and let the baked apple slices cool slightly.
- Sprinkle chopped pecans or walnuts over the baked apple slices if desired.
- Drizzle honey over the top for added sweetness if desired.
- Serve warm and enjoy these delicious and comforting baked apple slices with cinnamon!

Health Benefits:

- Apples are low in potassium and provide fiber, vitamins, and antioxidants, supporting digestive health and immune function.

- Cinnamon adds warmth and flavor and may help regulate blood sugar levels, promoting metabolic health.

- Nuts provide healthy fats and protein, promoting heart health and satiety.

Nutritional Value (per serving):

- Calories: 120

- Protein: 1g

- Carbohydrates: 20g

- Fat: 5g

- Fiber: 4g

- Potassium: 150mg

Preparation Time: 30 minutes

8: Lemon Yogurt Parfait with Almond Crunch

Ingredients:

- 1/2 cup plain Greek yogurt (low-fat)

- Zest of 1 lemon

- 1 tablespoon lemon juice

- 1 tablespoon honey

- 1/4 cup granola (low-sugar)

- 1 tablespoon sliced almonds

Instructions:

- In a small bowl, mix the plain Greek yogurt with lemon zest, lemon juice, and honey until well combined.
- In a serving glass or bowl, layer the lemon yogurt mixture with granola and sliced almonds.
- Repeat the layers until all ingredients are used, ending with a layer of granola and sliced almonds on top.
- Serve immediately and enjoy this refreshing and tangy lemon yogurt parfait with almond crunch!

Health Benefits:

- Greek yogurt is a good source of protein and calcium, promoting muscle health and bone health.
- Lemon provides vitamin C and antioxidants, supporting immune function and skin health.
- Granola and sliced almonds add texture and provide healthy fats and fiber, promoting satiety and digestive health.

Nutritional Value (per serving):

- Calories: 180
- Protein: 8g
- Carbohydrates: 20g
- Fat: 7g
- Fiber: 3g

- Potassium: 200mg

Preparation Time: 5 minutes

9: Berry Compote with Coconut Cream

Ingredients:

- 1 cup mixed berries (such as strawberries, blueberries, and raspberries), fresh or frozen
- 1 tablespoon honey or maple syrup
- 1/2 teaspoon vanilla extract
- 1/4 cup unsweetened coconut cream

Instructions:

- In a saucepan, combine the mixed berries, honey or maple syrup, and vanilla extract.
- Cook over medium heat, stirring occasionally, until the berries start to break down and release their juices, about 5-7 minutes.
- Remove from heat and let the berry compote cool slightly.
- Divide the berry compote into serving bowls or glasses.
- Top each serving with a dollop of unsweetened coconut cream.
- Serve warm or chilled, and enjoy this vibrant and fruity berry compote with coconut cream!

Health Benefits:

- Berries are low in potassium and provide fiber, vitamins, and antioxidants, supporting heart health and cognitive function.
- Honey or maple syrup adds natural sweetness and provides antioxidants and antimicrobial properties, promoting overall health and well-being.
- Coconut cream provides healthy fats and adds creaminess without dairy, making it suitable for individuals with lactose intolerance or dairy allergies.

Nutritional Value (per serving):

- Calories: 100
- Protein: 1g
- Carbohydrates: 15g
- Fat: 5g
- Fiber: 4g
- Potassium: 150mg

Preparation Time: 10 minutes

10: Frozen Banana Bites

Ingredients:

- 2 ripe bananas, peeled and cut into bite-sized pieces
- 1/4 cup unsweetened almond butter or peanut butter

- 1/4 cup dark chocolate chips
- 2 tablespoons chopped nuts (such as almonds, walnuts, or pecans)

Instructions:

- Line a baking sheet with parchment paper.
- Spread almond butter or peanut butter on one side of each banana piece.
- Arrange the banana pieces in a single layer on the prepared baking sheet.
- Place the baking sheet in the freezer and freeze the banana bites for at least 1 hour, or until firm.
- In a microwave-safe bowl, melt the dark chocolate chips in 30-second intervals, stirring in between, until smooth and melted.
- Remove the frozen banana bites from the freezer.
- Using a fork, dip each banana bite into the melted chocolate, coating it halfway.
- Place the chocolate-coated banana bites back on the baking sheet.
- Sprinkle chopped nuts over the chocolate-coated side of each banana bite.

- Return the baking sheet to the freezer and freeze the banana bites for an additional 30 minutes, or until the chocolate is set.
- Serve chilled, and enjoy these delightful and satisfying frozen banana bites as a guilt-free dessert!

Health Benefits:

- Bananas are low in potassium and provide fiber, vitamins, and minerals, supporting digestive health and heart health.
- Almond butter or peanut butter provides healthy fats and protein, promoting satiety and supporting brain health.
- Dark chocolate contains antioxidants and may have heart-healthy benefits when consumed in moderation.

Nutritional Value (per serving):

- Calories: 150
- Protein: 3g
- Carbohydrates: 20g
- Fat: 8g
- Fiber: 4g
- Potassium: 200mg

Preparation Time: 20 minutes (plus freezing time)

CKD STAGE 4 SOUP RECIPES FOR SENIORS

1: Vegetable Quinoa Soup

Ingredients:

- 1 tablespoon olive oil
- 1 onion, chopped
- 2 carrots, diced
- 2 celery stalks, diced
- 2 cloves garlic, minced
- 1 teaspoon dried thyme
- 1/2 cup quinoa, rinsed
- 4 cups low-sodium vegetable broth
- 1 cup diced tomatoes (canned or fresh)
- 2 cups chopped spinach or kale
- Salt and pepper to taste
- Fresh parsley for garnish (optional)

Instructions:

- In a large pot, heat olive oil over medium heat. Add chopped onion, carrots, and celery. Cook until vegetables are softened, about 5-7 minutes.
- Add minced garlic and dried thyme to the pot. Cook for another 1-2 minutes until fragrant.

- Stir in rinsed quinoa, vegetable broth, and diced tomatoes. Bring the soup to a boil, then reduce heat to low and simmer for 15-20 minutes, or until quinoa is cooked and vegetables are tender.
- Add chopped spinach or kale to the soup during the last 5 minutes of cooking.
- Season with salt and pepper to taste.
- Ladle the vegetable quinoa soup into bowls, garnish with fresh parsley if desired, and serve hot.
- Enjoy this nutritious and hearty soup as a comforting meal!

Health Benefits:

- Quinoa is a complete protein and provides essential amino acids, making it an excellent source of plant-based protein for individuals with CKD Stage 4.
- Vegetables like carrots, celery, and spinach/kale are low in potassium and rich in vitamins, minerals, and antioxidants, supporting overall health and kidney function.
- Vegetable broth provides hydration and flavor without added sodium, making it suitable for individuals with CKD.

Nutritional Value (per serving):

- Calories: 180
- Protein: 5g

- Carbohydrates: 30g

- Fat: 5g

- Fiber: 5g

- Potassium: 400mg

Preparation Time: 30 minutes

2: Lentil and Vegetable Soup

Ingredients:

- 1 tablespoon olive oil

- 1 onion, chopped

- 2 carrots, diced

- 2 celery stalks, diced

- 2 cloves garlic, minced

- 1 cup dried green or brown lentils, rinsed

- 4 cups low-sodium vegetable broth

- 1 bay leaf

- 1 teaspoon ground cumin

- 1/2 teaspoon paprika

- Salt and pepper to taste

- Fresh parsley for garnish (optional)

Instructions: In a large pot, heat olive oil over medium heat. Add chopped onion, carrots, and celery. Cook until vegetables are softened, about 5-7 minutes.

- Add minced garlic to the pot and cook for another 1-2 minutes until fragrant.
- Stir in rinsed lentils, vegetable broth, bay leaf, ground cumin, and paprika. Bring the soup to a boil, then reduce heat to low and simmer for 20-25 minutes, or until lentils are tender.
- Season with salt and pepper to taste.
- Remove the bay leaf from the soup before serving.
- Ladle the lentil and vegetable soup into bowls, garnish with fresh parsley if desired, and serve hot.
- Enjoy this protein-packed and flavorful soup as a nutritious meal!

Health Benefits:

- Lentils are high in protein, fiber, and iron, making them an excellent plant-based protein source for individuals with CKD Stage 4.
- Carrots, celery, and onions provide vitamins, minerals, and antioxidants, supporting overall health and kidney function.
- Spices like cumin and paprika add flavor without added sodium, enhancing the taste of the soup.

Nutritional Value (per serving):

- Calories: 200

- Protein: 10g

- Carbohydrates: 30g

- Fat: 5g

- Fiber: 10g

- Potassium: 350mg

Preparation Time: 40 minutes

3: Mushroom Barley Soup

Ingredients:

- 1 tablespoon olive oil

- 1 onion, chopped

- 2 carrots, diced

- 2 celery stalks, diced

- 8 ounces mushrooms, sliced

- 2 cloves garlic, minced

- 1/2 cup pearl barley, rinsed

- 4 cups low-sodium vegetable broth

- 1 bay leaf

- 1 teaspoon dried thyme

- Salt and pepper to taste

- Fresh parsley for garnish (optional)

Instructions:

- In a large pot, heat olive oil over medium heat. Add chopped onion, carrots, and celery. Cook until vegetables are softened, about 5-7 minutes.
- Add sliced mushrooms to the pot and cook until they release their juices and start to brown, about 5 minutes.
- Add minced garlic and cook for another 1-2 minutes until fragrant.
- Stir in rinsed pearl barley, vegetable broth, bay leaf, and dried thyme. Bring the soup to a boil, then reduce heat to low and simmer for 30-35 minutes, or until barley is tender.
- Season with salt and pepper to taste.
- Remove the bay leaf from the soup before serving.
- Ladle the mushroom barley soup into bowls, garnish with fresh parsley if desired, and serve hot.
- Enjoy this hearty and satisfying soup as a nutritious meal!

Health Benefits:

- Barley is high in fiber and may help regulate blood sugar levels and promote heart health.
- Mushrooms provide umami flavor and are low in potassium, making them suitable for individuals with CKD Stage 4.
- Thyme adds aroma and flavor and may have antibacterial and anti-inflammatory properties.

Nutritional Value (per serving):

- Calories: 200
- Protein: 6g
- Carbohydrates: 35g
- Fat: 4g
- Fiber: 8g
- Potassium: 300mg

Preparation Time: 45 minutes

4: Red Lentil Soup with Spinach

Ingredients:

- 1 tablespoon olive oil
- 1 onion, chopped
- 2 carrots, diced
- 2 celery stalks, diced
- 2 cloves garlic, minced
- 1 cup dried red lentils, rinsed
- 4 cups low-sodium vegetable broth
- 1 teaspoon ground cumin
- 1/2 teaspoon ground coriander
- 2 cups chopped spinach
- Juice of 1 lemon
- Salt and pepper to taste

- Fresh cilantro for garnish (optional)

Instructions:

- In a large pot, heat olive oil over medium heat. Add chopped onion, carrots, and celery. Cook until vegetables are softened, about 5-7 minutes.
- Add minced garlic and cook for another 1-2 minutes until fragrant.
- Stir in rinsed red lentils, vegetable broth, ground cumin, and ground coriander. Bring the soup to a boil, then reduce heat to low and simmer for 20-25 minutes, or until lentils are tender.
- Add chopped spinach to the pot and cook for another 5 minutes until wilted.
- Stir in lemon juice and season with salt and pepper to taste.
- Ladle the red lentil soup into bowls, garnish with fresh cilantro if desired, and serve hot.
- Enjoy this flavorful and nutritious soup as a comforting meal!

Health Benefits:

- Red lentils are rich in protein and fiber, supporting digestive health and providing sustained energy.

- Spinach is low in potassium and provides vitamins, minerals, and antioxidants, promoting overall health and kidney function.

- Lemon juice adds brightness and may aid digestion and detoxification.

Nutritional Value (per serving):

- Calories: 180

- Protein: 8g

- Carbohydrates: 30g

- Fat: 4g

- Fiber: 8g

- Potassium: 250mg

Preparation Time: 40 minutes

5: Cauliflower and Leek Soup

Ingredients:

- 1 tablespoon olive oil

- 2 leeks, white and light green parts only, sliced

- 1 head cauliflower, chopped

- 2 cloves garlic, minced

- 4 cups low-sodium vegetable broth

- 1 teaspoon dried thyme

- 1/2 teaspoon ground turmeric
- Salt and pepper to taste
- Fresh chives for garnish (optional)

Instructions:

- In a large pot, heat olive oil over medium heat. Add sliced leeks and cook until softened, about 5 minutes.
- Add chopped cauliflower and minced garlic to the pot. Cook for another 3-4 minutes until cauliflower begins to soften.
- Pour in vegetable broth and add dried thyme and ground turmeric. Bring the soup to a boil, then reduce heat to low and simmer for 20-25 minutes, or until cauliflower is tender.
- Use an immersion blender or transfer the soup to a blender and blend until smooth.
- Season with salt and pepper to taste.
- Ladle the cauliflower and leek soup into bowls, garnish with fresh chives if desired, and serve hot.
- Enjoy this creamy and flavorful soup as a comforting meal!

Health Benefits:

- Cauliflower is low in potassium and provides vitamins C and K, fiber, and antioxidants, supporting overall health and kidney function.

- Leeks add a mild onion flavor and are low in potassium, making them suitable for individuals with CKD Stage 4.

- Turmeric has anti-inflammatory properties and may help reduce oxidative stress.

Nutritional Value (per serving):

- Calories: 150

- Protein: 5g

- Carbohydrates: 20g

- Fat: 7g

- Fiber: 5g

- Potassium: 300mg

Preparation Time: 35 minutes

6: White Bean and Kale Soup

Ingredients:

- 1 tablespoon olive oil

- 1 onion, chopped

- 2 carrots, diced

- 2 celery stalks, diced

- 2 cloves garlic, minced

- 2 cans (15 ounces each) white beans, drained and rinsed

- 4 cups low-sodium vegetable broth

- 2 cups chopped kale
- 1 teaspoon dried rosemary
- 1/2 teaspoon smoked paprika
- Salt and pepper to taste
- Fresh parsley for garnish (optional)

Instructions:

- In a large pot, heat olive oil over medium heat. Add chopped onion, carrots, and celery. Cook until vegetables are softened, about 5-7 minutes.
- Add minced garlic to the pot and cook for another 1-2 minutes until fragrant.
- Stir in drained and rinsed white beans, vegetable broth, dried rosemary, and smoked paprika. Bring the soup to a boil, then reduce heat to low and simmer for 15-20 minutes.
- Add chopped kale to the pot and cook for another 5 minutes until wilted.
- Season with salt and pepper to taste.
- Ladle the white bean and kale soup into bowls, garnish with fresh parsley if desired, and serve hot.
- Enjoy this hearty and nutritious soup as a satisfying meal!

Health Benefits: White beans are a good source of plant-based protein and fiber, supporting digestive health and providing long-lasting energy.

- Kale is low in potassium and rich in vitamins A, C, and K, calcium, and antioxidants, promoting overall health and kidney function.
- Rosemary and smoked paprika add depth of flavor and may have antioxidant and anti-inflammatory properties.

Nutritional Value (per serving):

- Calories: 220
- Protein: 10g
- Carbohydrates: 30g
- Fat: 5g
- Fiber: 10g
- Potassium: 400mg

Preparation Time: 40 minutes

5: Butternut Squash and Apple Soup

Ingredients:

- 1 butternut squash, peeled, seeded, and cubed
- 2 apples, peeled, cored, and chopped
- 1 onion, chopped
- 2 cloves garlic, minced
- 4 cups low-sodium vegetable broth
- 1 teaspoon ground cinnamon

- 1/2 teaspoon ground nutmeg

- Salt and pepper to taste

- 1 tablespoon olive oil

- Fresh sage leaves for garnish (optional)

Instructions:

1. In a large pot, heat olive oil over medium heat. Add chopped onion and cook until softened, about 5 minutes.

2. Add minced garlic and cook for another 1-2 minutes until fragrant.

3. Add cubed butternut squash and chopped apples to the pot. Cook for 5 minutes, stirring occasionally.

4. Pour in vegetable broth and bring the mixture to a boil. Reduce heat to low and simmer for 20-25 minutes, or until the squash and apples are tender.

5. Using an immersion blender or regular blender, puree the soup until smooth.

6. Stir in ground cinnamon and ground nutmeg. Season with salt and pepper to taste.

7. Ladle the butternut squash and apple soup into bowls, garnish with fresh sage leaves if desired, and serve hot.

8. Enjoy this comforting and flavorful soup as a nutritious meal!

Health Benefits:

- Butternut squash and apples are low in potassium and high in vitamins, minerals, and antioxidants, supporting kidney health and overall well-being.
- Cinnamon and nutmeg add warmth and sweetness without added sugar, enhancing the flavor of the soup.

Nutritional Value (per serving):

- Calories: 150
- Protein: 2g
- Carbohydrates: 35g
- Fat: 2g
- Fiber: 6g
- Potassium: 300mg

Preparation Time: 40 minutes

6: Creamy Cauliflower Soup

Ingredients:

- 1 cauliflower head, chopped into florets
- 1 onion, chopped
- 2 cloves garlic, minced
- 4 cups low-sodium vegetable broth

- 1/2 cup unsweetened almond milk (or low-fat milk for non-vegan option)
- 1 tablespoon olive oil
- Salt and pepper to taste
- Fresh chives for garnish (optional)

Instructions:

- In a large pot, heat olive oil over medium heat. Add chopped onion and cook until softened, about 5 minutes.
- Add minced garlic and cook for another 1-2 minutes until fragrant.
- Add cauliflower florets to the pot and sauté for 5 minutes, stirring occasionally.
- Pour in vegetable broth and bring the mixture to a boil. Reduce heat to low and simmer for 20-25 minutes, or until the cauliflower is tender.
- Using an immersion blender or regular blender, puree the soup until smooth.
- Stir in unsweetened almond milk (or low-fat milk) to achieve desired creaminess. Season with salt and pepper to taste.
- Ladle the creamy cauliflower soup into bowls, garnish with fresh chives if desired, and serve hot.
- Enjoy this velvety and satisfying soup as a comforting meal!

Health Benefits:

- Cauliflower is low in potassium and high in fiber, providing digestive support and promoting heart health.
- Almond milk adds creaminess without added dairy, making the soup suitable for individuals with lactose intolerance.
- Garlic and onion add flavor and may have anti-inflammatory properties, supporting overall health.

Nutritional Value (per serving):

- Calories: 120
- Protein: 4g
- Carbohydrates: 20g
- Fat: 4g
- Fiber: 6g
- Potassium: 250mg

Preparation Time: 35 minutes

7: Lemon Chicken Vegetable Soup

Ingredients:

- 1 tablespoon olive oil
- 1 onion, chopped
- 2 carrots, diced
- 2 celery stalks, diced

- 2 cloves garlic, minced
- 6 cups low-sodium chicken broth
- 2 cups cooked chicken breast, shredded
- 1 cup green beans, trimmed and chopped
- 1 zucchini, diced
- Juice of 1 lemon
- 1 teaspoon dried thyme
- Salt and pepper to taste
- Fresh parsley for garnish (optional)

Instructions:

- In a large pot, heat olive oil over medium heat. Add chopped onion, carrots, and celery. Cook until vegetables are softened, about 5-7 minutes.
- Add minced garlic and cook for another 1-2 minutes until fragrant.
- Pour in chicken broth and bring the mixture to a boil.
- Add shredded chicken breast, chopped green beans, diced zucchini, lemon juice, and dried thyme to the pot. Reduce heat to low and simmer for 15-20 minutes, or until vegetables are tender.
- Season with salt and pepper to taste.
- Ladle the lemon chicken vegetable soup into bowls, garnish with fresh parsley if desired, and serve hot.

- Enjoy this comforting and nourishing soup as a wholesome meal!

Health Benefits:

- Chicken provides lean protein and essential nutrients, supporting muscle health and immune function.
- Green beans and zucchini are low in potassium and high in fiber, vitamins, and minerals, promoting digestive health and overall well-being.
- Lemon juice adds brightness and flavor without added sodium, enhancing the taste of the soup.

Nutritional Value (per serving):

- Calories: 200
- Protein: 20g
- Carbohydrates: 15g
- Fat: 6g
- Fiber: 4g
- Potassium: 350mg

Preparation Time: 30 minutes

8: Lentil and Vegetable Soup

Ingredients:

- 1 tablespoon olive oil

- 1 onion, chopped
- 2 carrots, diced
- 2 celery stalks, diced
- 2 cloves garlic, minced
- 1 cup dried green or brown lentils, rinsed
- 6 cups low-sodium vegetable broth
- 1 teaspoon ground cumin
- 1/2 teaspoon smoked paprika
- 1 bay leaf
- Salt and pepper to taste
- Fresh cilantro for garnish (optional)

Instructions:

- In a large pot, heat olive oil over medium heat. Add chopped onion, carrots, and celery. Cook until vegetables are softened, about 5-7 minutes.
- Add minced garlic and cook for another 1-2 minutes until fragrant.
- Stir in rinsed lentils, vegetable broth, ground cumin, smoked paprika, and bay leaf. Bring the soup to a boil, then reduce heat to low and simmer for 25-30 minutes, or until lentils are tender.
- Season with salt and pepper to taste.

- Ladle the lentil and vegetable soup into bowls, garnish with fresh cilantro if desired, and serve hot.
- Enjoy this hearty and satisfying soup as a nutritious meal!

Health Benefits:

- Lentils are a good source of plant-based protein and fiber, supporting satiety and digestive health.
- Carrots and celery provide vitamins, minerals, and antioxidants, promoting immune function and cellular health.
- Cumin and smoked paprika add depth of flavor and may have anti-inflammatory properties, supporting overall well-being.

Nutritional Value (per serving):

- Calories: 220
- Protein: 14g
- Carbohydrates: 30g
- Fat: 4g
- Fiber: 10g
- Potassium: 400mg

Preparation Time: 40 minutes

Ingredients:

- 1 tablespoon olive oil
- 1 onion, chopped
- 2 cloves garlic, minced
- 4 cups low-sodium vegetable broth
- 4 cups diced tomatoes (fresh or canned)
- 1/4 cup tomato paste
- 1 teaspoon dried basil
- 1/2 teaspoon dried oregano
- Salt and pepper to taste
- Fresh basil leaves for garnish (optional)

Instructions:

- In a large pot, heat olive oil over medium heat. Add chopped onion and cook until softened, about 5 minutes.
- Add minced garlic and cook for another 1-2 minutes until fragrant.
- Stir in diced tomatoes, tomato paste, dried basil, and dried oregano. Cook for 5 minutes, allowing the flavors to meld together.
- Pour in vegetable broth and bring the mixture to a boil. Reduce heat to low and simmer for 20-25 minutes.

- Using an immersion blender or regular blender, puree the soup until smooth.
- Season with salt and pepper to taste.
- Ladle the tomato basil soup into bowls, garnish with fresh basil leaves if desired, and serve hot.
- Enjoy this classic and comforting soup as a flavorful meal!

Health Benefits:

- Tomatoes are rich in lycopene, a powerful antioxidant that may help reduce inflammation and protect against chronic diseases.
- Basil adds a burst of freshness and flavor, enhancing the taste of the soup without added sodium.

Nutritional Value (per serving):

- Calories: 120
- Protein: 3g
- Carbohydrates: 20g
- Fat: 4g
- Fiber: 5g
- Potassium: 450mg

Preparation Time: 30 minutes

10: Spinach and White Bean Soup

Ingredients:

- 1 tablespoon olive oil

- 1 onion, chopped

- 2 cloves garlic, minced

- 4 cups low-sodium vegetable broth

- 2 cups chopped fresh spinach leaves

- 1 can (15 ounces) white beans, drained and rinsed

- 1 teaspoon dried thyme

- 1/2 teaspoon dried rosemary

- Salt and pepper to taste

- Fresh parsley for garnish (optional)

Instructions:

- In a large pot, heat olive oil over medium heat. Add chopped onion and cook until softened, about 5 minutes.

- Add minced garlic and cook for another 1-2 minutes until fragrant.

- Stir in chopped spinach leaves and cook until wilted, about 2-3 minutes.

- Add white beans, dried thyme, and dried rosemary to the pot. Cook for 5 minutes, allowing the flavors to meld together.

- Pour in vegetable broth and bring the mixture to a boil. Reduce heat to low and simmer for 15-20 minutes.

- Season with salt and pepper to taste.

- Ladle the spinach and white bean soup into bowls, garnish with fresh parsley if desired, and serve hot.

- Enjoy this nutritious and satisfying soup as a wholesome meal!

Health Benefits:

- Spinach is packed with vitamins, minerals, and antioxidants, supporting overall health and kidney function.

- White beans are high in protein and fiber, helping to stabilize blood sugar levels and promote satiety.

Nutritional Value (per serving):

- Calories: 180

- Protein: 9g

- Carbohydrates: 25g

- Fat: 5g

- Fiber: 8g

- Potassium: 350mg

Preparation Time: 35 minutes

CONCLUSION

This CKD Stage 4 Cookbook for Seniors serves as a comprehensive guide and valuable resource for individuals navigating the challenges of chronic kidney disease. With a focus on nourishing and kidney-friendly recipes, this cookbook aims to empower seniors with the knowledge and tools they need to support their health and well-being.

Throughout this cookbook, we've provided a diverse selection of recipes that are not only delicious but also tailored to the specific dietary needs of individuals with CKD Stage 4. From nutritious breakfast options to hearty soups and satisfying desserts, each recipe has been carefully crafted to be both flavorful and supportive of kidney health.

In addition to providing mouthwatering recipes, this cookbook also offers valuable information on understanding CKD Stage 4, managing symptoms, and making lifestyle modifications to support kidney function. From tips on selecting fresh produce to guidance on portion control and meal planning, we've strived to equip seniors with the knowledge and tools they need to take control of their health.

As we conclude this cookbook, we encourage seniors with CKD Stage 4 to embrace the power of nutrition and make positive changes to their diet and lifestyle.

By incorporating kidney-friendly foods and adopting healthy habits, seniors can take proactive steps towards managing their condition, preventing complications, and improving their overall quality of life.

We hope that this cookbook serves as a valuable companion on your journey to better health and well-being. Remember, each recipe is not just a meal but a step towards a healthier future. Let's continue to nourish our bodies, support our kidneys, and thrive at every stage of life

www.ingramcontent.com/pod-product-compliance
Lightning Source LLC
Chambersburg PA
CBHW050824260726